# Public Health, Personal Health and Pills

T0199400

*Public Health, Personal Health and Pills* explores the processes and effects of the increasing governance of our lives through pharmaceuticals, looking at the moral, interactional, social and political forces that shape our use of them. It demonstrates the ways in which social relationships and identities are developed, sustained and transformed through medication use.

Building on the extensive medicalisation of health literature, and the more recent concept of pharmaceuticalisation, this pioneering book is firmly based on empirical research and sociological theory. It brings together macro considerations of trends in pharmaceutical consumption, regulation and policy, micro considerations of the decision-making and the negotiation of medication use in homes and clinics, and an institutional analysis of the role of drug monitoring agencies, drug subsidising agencies, drug trial methodologies and the media.

This book is a contribution to a burgeoning sociological interest in medication use, and will be of interest to a multidisciplinary audience of scholars and students of sociology, science and technology studies, pharmacy and health studies.

**Kevin Dew** is a Professor of Sociology at Victoria University of Wellington, New Zealand. He is a founding member of the Applied Research on Communication in Health (ARCH) Group. Current research activities include studies of interactions between health professionals and patients, cancer care decision-making in relation to health inequities and the social meanings of medications.

# Routledge Studies in the Sociology of Health and Illness

www.routledge.com/Routledge-Studies-in-the-Sociology-of-Health-and-Illness/book-series/RSSHI

# Public Health, Personal Health and Pills

Drug Entanglements and Pharmaceuticalised Governance

**Kevin Dew**

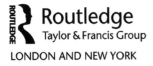

Routledge
Taylor & Francis Group

LONDON AND NEW YORK

First published 2019 by Routledge

2 Park Square, Milton Park, Abingdon, Oxfordshire OX14 4RN
52 Vanderbilt Avenue, New York, NY 10017

*Routledge is an imprint of the Taylor & Francis Group, an informa business*

First issued in paperback 2019

Copyright © 2019 Kevin Dew

The right of Kevin Dew to be identified as author of this work has been asserted by him in accordance with sections 77 and 78 of the Copyright, Designs and Patents Act 1988.

All rights reserved. No part of this book may be reprinted or reproduced or utilised in any form or by any electronic, mechanical, or other means, now known or hereafter invented, including photocopying and recording, or in any information storage or retrieval system, without permission in writing from the publishers.

Notice:
Product or corporate names may be trademarks or registered trademarks, and are used only for identification and explanation without intent to infringe.

*British Library Cataloguing-in-Publication Data*
A catalogue record for this book is available from the British Library

*Library of Congress Cataloging-in-Publication Data*
Names: Dew, Kevin, author.
Title: Public health, personal health and pills : drug entanglements and pharmaceuticalised governance / Kevin Dew.
Other titles: Routledge studies in the sociology of health and illness.
Description: Abingdon, Oxon ; New York, NY : Routledge, 2018. |
Series: Routledge studies in the sociology of health and illness | Includes bibliographical references and index.
Identifiers: LCCN 2018014833 | ISBN 9781138229389 (hardback) | ISBN 9781315389684 (ebook)
Subjects: | MESH: Prescription Drugs–therapeutic use | Drug Therapy–psychology | Attitude to Health | Prescription Drugs–adverse effects | Drug Industry | Pharmacovigilance
Classification: LCC RA401.A3 | NLM QV 55 | DDC 338.4/76151–dc23
LC record available at https://lccn.loc.gov/2018014833

ISBN: 978-1-138-22938-9 (hbk)
ISBN: 978-0-367-45753-2 (pbk)

Typeset in Times New Roman
by Wearset Ltd, Boldon, Tyne and Wear

# Contents

# Acknowledgements

My sincere thanks to all of my colleagues whose input has contributed to this book in so many ways. Amongst all those colleagues special thanks to Kerry Chamberlain, John Gardner, Jon Gabe, Darrin Hodgetts, Helen Madden, Linda Nikora, Pauline Norris and Alan Radley from the social meanings of medication team, and Tony Dowell, Lindsay Macdonald, Libby Plumridge, Rachel Tester and Maria Stubbe from the Applied Research on Communication in Health Group, and Chris Cunningham, Cheryl Davies, Carolyn Hooper, Diana Sarfati, Louise Signal, Jeannine Stairmand and Helen Tavite from the C3 Cancer Research Group. I would also like to thank Josh Barton and Georgia Lockie for their very helpful comments and suggestions.

# 1 Orienting to pharmaceuticalised governance

Pharmaceuticals are not simply material objects that have physiological effects; they additionally carry symbolic weight and evoke emotional responses. How we relate to them is underpinned by our values and our sense of morality. They may symbolise hope for a cure or for the control of disabling symptoms, or they may symbolise a failure to cope without relying on chemical agents. Pharmaceuticals may evoke a sense of joy at the prospect of overcoming difficult circumstances or, in the case of psychotropic drugs, fear of losing control over one's mind and body.

We may view drugs as a right that all people should have access to or as a means by which drug companies can gouge out huge profits by preying on people's anxieties and vulnerabilities. We may see ourselves as having a responsibility to take medications prescribed by experts or as being responsible for avoiding medications unless they are absolutely necessary. Like other technologies, we might stand in a relationship of what Sarah Franklin calls technological ambivalence with pharmaceuticals (Franklin 2013: 25). The technology offers hope and opportunity, but may also cause damage. The technology is produced in order to make a profit for some, and save lives for others. The symbolic and moral underpinnings of medications are one means by which they come to govern us, to influence and shape our conduct, activities, behaviours and thoughts.

## Orientation

It is important to provide a sense of the orientation of this book to offer some pointers to the reader. As an instance of this orientation, the prior sentence can be unpacked a little. First, this book does not have an orientation in that the book is not a conscious thinking entity. It is me, the author, who has the orientation. I want to bring this conscious thinking author into the narrative, particularly in those places in the book that are firmly grounded in my own research or research that I have undertaken with others. By doing so, I hope to convey a sense of the processes of knowledge production, or my own pathways to understanding. Second, the opening sentence to this section suggests the possibility of one orientation, but this too can be challenged. The theoretical positioning taken in this book will vary according to what is being looked at. Different theories may have conflicting underlying assumptions, values, epistemologies and ontologies. These differences are not just to be ignored; the position I take is that there is not just one way of seeing and understanding the social world, and depending on what you are looking at, insight will be gained by drawing on different conceptual and analytic tools.

One of my orientations, then, is that I want to put some work in to exposing how I got to my own particular understandings. This hopefully provides the reader with an understanding of the contingent processes of knowledge production. This is done not to undermine the arguments being made, but perhaps to make them more convincing. That although I might stumble across interpretations, this is not done in a vacuum but is a process or reacting to my understanding of my own values and what I encounter in the social world.

This approach has been influenced by teaching an undergraduate course called 'Knowledge, Power and Social Research' at my university. In this course I have tried to get students to think about what enables and what constrains knowledge production, and what it is that we can know, or say. In undertaking this task, I have had the students consider broad, high level ways in which knowledge and understanding is shaped. For example, Foucault uses the term 'episteme' to refer to general forms of thinking and assumptions that establish, or set the parameters for, what ideas can appear and what can be credibly talked about (Foucault 1970). Weber refers to rationalising processes in society, where scientific and bureaucratic processes increasingly exclude traditional, experiential and charismatic forms of authority. Increasing rationality underlines transformations in institutions and social relationships in society (Albrow 1970). These are the sort of broad, high level ideas we would discuss in class.

Further, I ask students to consider the way in which disciplines shape understanding, and so we consider ways of thinking and practices that are allowed in our own discipline of sociology. We have discussed how different methodologies shape what it is you come to see and understand, very broadly under the division of positivism and approaches that contest positivism. We consider the way our own values and experiences shape or influence what it is we come to see, interpret and 'know'. Through teaching this course I have come to reflect more on my own processes of research and interpretation, and on the importance of challenging dominant views about knowledge production that, to me, present a very distorted idea of research and its findings.

To illustrate, one particular situation made me consider doing things differently. I was presenting a session to some students on the relationship between theory and research. Rather than discuss major debates about this, I wanted to show the students my own processes, thinking that this might help to demystify links between theory and data. I used some research on the social meanings of medications to do this.

As part of this session I presented the students with some slides linking, in a mutually interacting relationship, data with orienting concepts (Layder 1998) with interpretations, shown in Figure 1.1.

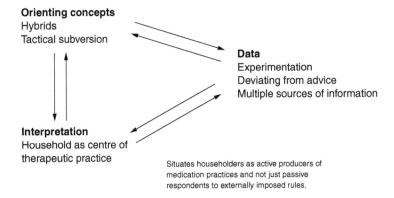

**Orienting concepts**
Hybrids
Tactical subversion

**Data**
Experimentation
Deviating from advice
Multiple sources of information

**Interpretation**
Household as centre of
therapeutic practice

Situates householders as active producers of
medication practices and not just passive
respondents to externally imposed rules.

*Figure 1.1* Diagram relating data, concepts and interpretations.

I explained how in research based on interviews with householders about their medication use (discussed more fully in Chapters 4 and 5), I came up with a number of codes and themes from the interview data, including themes of experimentation with medicines, deviating from the advice of health professionals and having multiple sources of information. I then told the students that, at the time, I had been reading a book by Anders Blok and Torben Jensen (2011) on the work of Bruno Latour, which included the concept of hybrids. I had encountered this concept many years before, but having come across it again I started to think how useful it would be in providing some insight into the household use of medications. From this interaction between the data and the orienting concept of hybrids, as well as other concepts I found useful, I came up with an interpretation: that households could be insightfully viewed as centres of therapeutic practice.

I told the students that I had written up this interpretation and that it had been published. One of the students raised his hand to ask me if, in the published journal article, I had noted how I arrived at the idea of using the concept of hybrids, that is, that I had just happened to be reading the book at the same time. I said of course not, because that is not what we do. That is not a convention of our discipline.

That interaction brought me up short. I now started to question why we do not expose how we come to our understandings. I got a strong sense that we are forced into presenting a false image of our work processes if we want to be published, and that gives a false sense of how the world is understood. I want to try to get a bit closer to how it is that we come to understand the world, with the view that through this we are in a better position to respond to and act on the world. In parallel, chapters in this book will explore how the pharmaceutical industry and others present a particular image of their work processes, which are perhaps distorted in ways that have real consequences for us all.

## Impacts of experiences

In the following, I outline some of the important moments in my experiential and intellectual biography, the sort of moments that influence how I see and interpret the social world, which includes the understandings I have arrived at in relation to pharmaceuticals.

After completing my first degree, a BA in Sociology and Psychology, I travelled from New Zealand to England and decided to study osteopathy. Encountering the world of an 'alternative' or 'complementary' medicine and exploring it in some depth shaped my way of thinking about pharmaceuticals; I was introduced to the idea that a medication-based therapeutics was not all it was made out to be. I encountered a number of ideas for the first time. One idea was that treating the symptoms with drugs is not treating the cause of the problem and it is better to focus on the cause. Another was that suppressing symptoms with medications might make things worse for the patient in the long run as an acute problem could be transformed into a chronic one. The view that there were other ways of treating people that had both empirical and theoretical support that was non-drug-based was prominent. As a good student, I took these and other ideas seriously and attempted to apply them.

Whilst studying I encountered circumstances that have stayed with me and fired my desire to understand how we think and how we give credibility to different understandings of the world, a desire that eventually led me back to sociology after completing my osteopathic training and spending a number of years in osteopathic clinics. One of these encounters I would like to unpack in a little detail.

I was training at an osteopathic school where, in my opinion and in the opinion of many other students, the principal had some exceptional skills in physical manipulation. The school was small and had not been going for long, and employed some teachers who had trained at another osteopathic school, which has a very biomedical focus. One day during a supervised student clinic, a man who had very intense back pain and could not support his own weight was carried in by his workmates. The principal of the college brought the man into his treatment room and a number of students and teachers gathered around, including me. The principal treated the man, and as part of the treatment he performed what was called a sacroiliac adjustment. This produced the standard 'clicking' sound and the man was immediately relieved of his pain, and was able to walk out of the clinic afterwards. Some of us students commented on this, along the lines that we would love to be as proficient as the principal and deal with acute problems in such a way. The teachers who had trained at the school that had embraced biomedical philosophies took a different view. They did not believe that the principal had actually done anything and explained the sudden recovery of the man as being the result of spontaneous recovery or an outcome of a placebo effect. They were trained in such a way that the type of manipulation the principal did was not given any credibility as it had not passed the required scientific test of a randomised controlled trial. There was then, for them, no evidence that it worked.

At the time I could not comprehend the teachers' response. We had all witnessed the same event, but we had come to completely different interpretations. How could that be? We can consider a number of explanations. The students and teachers were trained in different ways. They were operating with a different set of constructs about what was and was not possible. The students and teachers had different views on what was legitimate knowledge or legitimate evidence. Were the teachers and students operating within different paradigms, or thought collectives, which meant that for the teachers the treatment outcome was an anomaly that needed to be explained away, but for the students this was a perfectly expected outcome?

The concepts of paradigms and thought collectives were concepts I encountered after I had returned to sociology to undertake postgraduate studies. The term paradigm comes from a well-known book written by Thomas Kuhn (1970), *The Structure of Scientific Revolutions*. Kuhn, an historian of science and a physicist, argued that science was a social institution and therefore was impacted by social influences like any other institution. Scientists are socialised, and through socialisation they come to behave in particular ways and take on certain sets of assumptions and values. Scientists learn the rules of their community. Ideas about what is right and wrong become fixed and so certain ways of doing things and certain ways of speaking are seen as proper and right. This general framework that scientists come to work within, with its unexamined assumptions shared by the community, is what Kuhn called a paradigm. When we operate within one paradigm we cannot, at the same time, see the world from another paradigm. A classic example of this is the incompatibility of the perspectives on the structure of the solar system of the Ptolemaic and Copernican paradigms respectively; the former sees the earth at the centre of the solar system, whilst the latter sees the sun at the centre of the solar system. We either see one or the other.

Thought collectives, a similar concept, was developed much earlier by Ludwig Fleck in his book *The Genesis of a Scientific Fact* originally written in the 1930s. Fleck was a scientist with some acclaim, who worked in the research lab that developed the Wassermann reaction for the detection of syphilis. From his observations of how science worked, Fleck believed that science operated within 'thought collectives', a community that carried a particular thought style (Fleck 1979: 39). Some aspects that Fleck ascribed to thought collectives include contradictions being unthinkable, anomalies being unseen and exceptions being explained away. Our habitual way of thinking comes to be seen as natural and the only one possible. So with my example of the sacroiliac adjustment it can be argued that the students and the teachers inhabited different paradigms or different thought collectives and so were not able to understand each other's points of view.

In a nutshell, the encounter with the different perceptions of the results of a sacroiliac adjustment led me to a position that has been labelled social constructionism, and particularly to the idea that what we see is shaped, and maybe even determined, by the particular social, cultural and historical setting that we are in. Knowledge is contestable. So what I present in this book is contestable. I am not claiming that I have the last word on the matters discussed. I take the view that, ideally, I am participating in a dialogue with you as the reader and with those whose work I draw on and whose work I contest. I offer an understanding, and interpretation, and attempt to exhibit how I come to it so that you can decide how convinced you are by my claims to having some insight into the role of medications in society.

Briefly, social constructionism does not mean that the social, which could include social interests, educational forms, institutional arrangements, social conventions and so on, is the only thing that counts in the production of knowledge. Other aspects of the world are involved in knowledge production, most obviously the material substance of the world. However, from a social constructionist perspective the meaning of things and objects is not inherent to the thing or object (Harris 2008). The meaning we give to things and objects is derived from the social, whether that be the way in which objects are situated within particular stories we tell, or whether the meaning is indexed to the particular social situation in which the object is encountered. I take the position that the meaning of medications is not inherent in the particular pharmaceutical. The meaning of a pharmaceutical is not simply about the physiological response it causes, but relates to a whole host of issues, such as who prescribes it, who is responsible for consuming it, where it is consumed, how it fits in with other therapeutic practices, how it is produced, who pays for it and so on.

Another concern of social constructionism is how reality is produced through meanings and through interactions (Harris 2008). The reality of pharmaceuticals being viewed as the answer to health problems is produced through particular understandings that develop over time and that get reproduced every day in our interactions with health advisors, friends and family? To grasp how the reality of current pharmaceutical consumption has come into being we need to have some historical understanding of the development of the pharmaceutical industry, some understanding of the rise of the medical profession and its right to diagnose and prescribe, the process of the consultation where decisions are made about medication use, the kinds of narratives or discourses that are available to us that influence our decisions about how to respond to illness and so on.

With these considerations in mind, in this book I attempt to explore in various ways the relationship between the self, pharmaceuticals and power. One concept that I consider provides insight here is that of pharmaceuticalised governance. I will elaborate on this further throughout this book, but, in essence, pharmaceuticalised governance refers to the routines of pharmaceutical consumption that are embedded in relations of power and domination. The relations of power and domination have specific consequences that require us to act and present ourselves in particular ways. The power that requires our conformity works through many means, such as the fear of stigma, the influence of marketing and the instigation of state polices that both constrain and enable what we can do in relation to pharmaceuticals.

I came to the concept of pharmaceuticalised governance through research on the moral meanings of medications. The term 'governance' signals the genealogy of this concept as an offspring of my encounter with the work of Michel Foucault. Foucault uses the term governmentality to refer to the 'contact between the technologies of domination of others and those of the self' (Foucault 1988: 19). Domination can come from many sources, such as the state, corporations, households, workplaces and we are ourselves always implicated in processes of domination. Foucault uses a metaphor of networks to describe the operations of power. Power is diffuse and there are interconnections between institutions, peoples and processes. The linking of the conduct of the self to other institutions is what I find particularly useful in the term pharmaceuticalised governance. The following is an often quoted text from Foucault's work.

> Individuals effect a number of operations on their own bodies, souls, thoughts, conduct and way of being so as to transform themselves in order to attain a certain state of happiness, purity, wisdom, perfection or immortality.
>
> (Foucault 1988: 18)

In this book I seek to explore in various ways entanglements between our ways of being and pharmaceuticals. Pharmaceuticalised governance is a term I use to provide a particular sense of those entanglements.

The term pharmaceuticalised placed before governance references the recent scholarship on pharmaceuticalisation, which will be covered in Chapter 3. At its simplest, pharmaceuticalisation is a process that refers to the expansions of opportunities for, and practices of, pharmaceutical interventions on human beings (Williams *et al.* 2011). Hence, pharmaceuticalised governance refers to the ways those opportunities and practices shape our conduct and ways of being. What kinds of 'subjects', as in citizens participating in society, are possible through pharmaceuticals? In what ways are we subjected by other organisations, professionals and social demands to consume pharmaceuticals? In this book, I explore a range of ways in which pharmaceuticals shape us as subjects and shape broader social arrangements, such as how health professionals behave, and how health policy is influenced through pharmaceuticals.

The influences shaping particular forms of pharmaceuticalised governance are myriad. Johanne Collin usefully deploys Foucault's concept of dispositif in considering the transformative power of pharmaceuticals in society (Collin 2016). A dispositif is a strategy, strangely enough without a strategist, that is the outcome of the accumulated effects of institutions, professions, practices, understandings and ways of knowing. I perhaps would abandon the term strategy here, but the focus on an accumulating process entangling many social practices is one that I hope to give some sense of throughout this book.

## Excluding the placebo

Our belief in the value of pharmaceuticals is based on their capacity to provide therapeutic value. There is a well-known phenomenon whereby people can obtain therapeutic value from agents that have no known active ingredient, which we call the placebo effect. The word placebo means 'to please'. If people believe they are receiving something beneficial for their health, then their health may improve. There is some power inherent in ourselves that produces physiological change that is not directly related to the treatment. The placebo effect is estimated to have a 30 to 40 per cent success rate, but this will vary according to such things as the means of delivery (an injection produces a more powerful placebo effect), the manner of the practitioner (a caring and compassionate manner is supposed to increase the placebo effect), and the condition the patient is suffering from. In order to prove that a particular substance or treatment is effective, we have to prove that it is better than the placebo effect.

The research methodology of double-blind randomised controlled trials (RCTs) was developed to determine whether a drug improves upon the placebo effect. 'Double-blind' means that neither the patient nor the person giving the treatment should know whether the treatment is the real one or a fake one. If the person giving the agent knows it is the treatment and not the fake, they can produce a 'healing' or placebo effect of their own. Therefore, neither the patient nor the practitioner must know whether the treatment is real or fake.

The development of the RCT is the outcome of a complex process where we see an important shift in what we find credible. Prior to the development of RCTs, physicians placed much greater reliance on their theoretical education and their experience. The shift to an increased reliance on clinical trials is what I have termed clinical legibility (Dew 2012), following the arguments of James Scott about fiscal legibility. Scott (1998) argues that over many centuries there have been developments that render intelligible and legible social practices, like the exchange of goods and services that were once messy and opaque. This process of increasing legibility allows for greater oversight by organisations and institutions, such as the state that may be distant from where such social practices occur.

Scott provides an illustrative example from rural Malaysia. If you asked 'How far is it to the next village?' a likely response would be 'three rice cookings' (Scott 1998: 25). This sort of response is locally meaningful, as to provide a distance does not take into account the terrain and difficulty, so time and time based on localised understandings of time where there are no wristwatches, is locally meaningful. Local knowledge and local understandings are used, not something that can be easily translated on to a standardised map.

The state or a government is empowered in relation to citizens when there is the establishment of standardised maps of a territory, and standardisation of weights and measures. These facilitate such things as trade and the collection of taxes and rates. Prior to such standardisation the value of, for example, land would be left to local people making assessments, and the same would apply to the value and quality of the products produced on the land. To determine what land taxes can be collected requires good maps, and to trade the products of the land with ease requires some measure of the quality and quantity of the product. Through the standardisation of maps and measures it becomes much easier to administer the population.

By analogy, clinical legibility can be seen as a goal of many developments in medicine that attempt to overcome variability in diagnoses, diagnostic tests and treatment plans. There are a whole range of activities that we can identify here, including Quality Assurance (QA), Evidence-Based Medicine (EBM) and guideline developments. The goal of such systems is to make the often messy and opaque clinical practices more quantifiable: they can be granted with 'value' and priced, and therefore enabling more centralised control over clinical activities.

Processes of centralisation are facilitated through this transformation of complex phenomena into objects of quantification (Porter 1995). Just as the fiscal illegibility in Scott's example is an outcome of variation in the local, contingent practices of those who own and work the land, clinical illegibility (from the point of view of those who wish to determine whether clinical resources are being used efficiently) is the consequence of the often complex and idiosyncratic interactions between clinicians and patients. Theodore Porter (1995) makes evident that before clinical practice could be rendered legible the quantification and standardisation of many clinical practices had to occur: for example, doses of medication required standardisation. The development of standardising procedures relating to pharmaceuticals and the critical role of the clinical trial will be discussed in the following chapter.

## The patient's role

The role of the patient has so far been somewhat missing from this abstract discussion. The outcomes of patient consultations are embedded in these developments around the credibility of knowledge, but the patient too has their own particular role. This has changed dramatically over time, and in Chapters 4 and 5 we will see how the demarcation between patient and therapists is quite fuzzy. Sociologists have shifted their understanding of the role of patients over many decades. An early ground-breaking argument about the patient role was made by the famous American sociologist Talcott Parsons. Parsons' concept of the sick role, which he developed in the 1950s, positioned the patient as someone who is socialised into particular ways of behaving and acting. What was ground-breaking about this view at the time was Parsons' compelling argument that sickness was not simply a biological event; it was a social process as well. This view was a challenging one to the medical profession at the time, and gave impetus to a more critical approach in sociology of health and illness.

For Parsons, health is 'the state of optimum capacity of an individual for the effective performance of the roles and tasks for which he [*sic*] has been social-ized' (Parsons 1958). Therefore, illness is the incapacity of an individual to effectively perform social roles. Parsons developed the idea of the sick role, a role that we are socialised into which provides the institutional means (that is, through the medical encounter) to overcome the motivation to stay sick. Why would we want to stay sick? Parsons argued that illness may become accepted as an alternative to fulfilling our normal role obligations because of the strong appeal of the comforting nurturance of family. The institution of medicine is then, according to Parsons, not one just to cure ills, but it has an important social function in facilitating the fulfilment of role obligations.

Parsons identified a number of features of the sick role. One is that recovery depends upon a therapeutic process. In this sense it is not the patient but the therapeutic agent that is responsible for recovery. Illness, additionally, exempts the sick person from normal role obligations. The state of being exempt from fulfilling one's normal roles, such as being a worker or a student, must be seen as undesirable and the patient must try to get well. The legitimate way to get well is to seek help from competent agencies. The agencies that are given the legitimacy of being competent are medical professionals. In sum, patients are required to seek help from doctors and follow their advice so that the patient, in turn, can have their exemption from duties legitimated. The sick role acts as a form of social control because if the patient is not motivated to seek help then the patient will be seen as deviant in some way, such as being a malingerer. This labelling of the patient as deviant removes the patient from influencing others to act in the same way.

Parsons interpretation expands what is available for sociological investigation. Sickness is not just a biological process; it is in many important ways a social one. We are socialised into the institution of medicine; we learn our roles and how to adjust to the interactions that occur in consultations and that occur in the home and workplace when signs and symptoms of illness occur.

Parsons' perspective can be interpreted as a paternalistic view in which the medical profession dominates, and there have been many developments in thinking about the clinical encounter since Parsons wrote this, but the sick role is still an important concept with utility. Some sociological traditions may note the asymmetries in consultations between patients and clinicians but patients are also viewed as active agents in decision-making (Costello and Roberts 2001). From this perspective, patients do not simply passively follow the advice of health professionals. More recent scholarship, influenced by Foucault's work on neoliberalism, focuses on ways in which patients are made responsible for their health care decision-making and the cultural demands placed on them to be positive and strong willed (Steinberg 2015). This approach expands the extent of role obligations on patients beyond Parsons' view. Patients, as good citizens, are required to be active and responsible (Gabe *et al.* 2015).

In the medical arena itself there have been efforts to develop a more patient-centred medicine with the goal of shared decision-making in medical consultations. Shared decision-making is conceptualised as a scenario where both the clinician and the patient are involved in the decision-making process and information exchange (Pollard *et al.* 2015). As will be discussed in Chapters 4 and 5, the notion of a clear demarcation between patient and clinician is not one that is sustainable for many in terms of everyday practices related to medications.

The concept of the sick role indicates ways in which we conduct ourselves differently when we are in a state of illness or disease. The requirement to seek competent help and the desire to get better relate directly to pharmaceuticalised governance, in that the sick role is at least one way in which we enter into this different form of governance. Parsons' focus was on acute illness and illness that we recover from. Sociological considerations of chronic illness require different concepts, as in some chronic illness situations the patient will not be able to return to their usual roles.

Mike Bury coined the term biographical disruption to describe the changes that occur when one's life is disrupted by chronic illness. Being diagnosed and experiencing a chronic illness disrupts one's assumptions about the future, and behaviours of the chronically ill person and those around them change in response to the change in the chronically ill person's body. The disruption requires the ill person to draw on different resources to cope, and this can change relationships between the ill person and their family and friends (Bury 1982). Attempts to mitigate that disruption often lead to attempts to control the signs and symptoms of disease or to prevent future deterioration of the body through medicines. These in turn require new ways of conducting oneself and changing one's relations with others and with therapeutic agents, such as pharmaceuticals. Pharmaceuticalised governance takes different forms, observed in the different responses to acute and chronic illness.

## What you will find

Throughout this book, you will encounter opposing positions on topics. There will be discussion about regulating the drug industry that is opposed by those who see this as restricting innovation and quick access to beneficial drugs. There will be discussion of potential patients having the right to whatever information drug companies wish to impart that is opposed by those who see drug companies manipulating people into consuming unnecessary drugs. There will be discussion about the state enforcing or promoting particular therapeutic practices, and the right for individuals to make their own choices. There will be discussion regarding the disclosure of information about such things as drug side effects and adverse reactions, with some insisting on full disclosure and others fearful that disclosure will scare people away from taking beneficial therapeutic approaches.

Very often people taking opposing positions can have the same goals, an overarching goal that we can all agree on, to improve the health of the population and relieve people from suffering. These opposing positions are then not always based on different goals, but different values and different understandings about how best to achieve those goals. Arguably some of these different understandings are based on principles. Drawing on the work of sociologist Vilfredo Pareto, Michael Billig suggests that principles need to be kept in check by countervailing forces or contrary principles (Billig 1996). He argues this based on his view that principles, expressed as simple formulations, are extremes and in these simplistic formulations cannot act as guides to social affairs. To simply illustrate we can take a commonly claimed principle, for example, the idea that the free market is the best way to organise the provision of goods and services. To argue this in the case of drugs, we could say that the person or company who has a life-saving drug should charge what they can get away with and that patients, or customers, will have to judge whether they can afford the cost or not. The principle of supply and demand rules. But this position can clash with countervailing forces, such as our sense of compassion for those facing terminal disease, or our sense of fairness for those who cannot afford to operate in this free market environment. With any principle there will be exceptions to any simple application that as a society or as a community we might insist on making. Billig refers to these kinds of contradictory forces as dilemmas of common sense, and the application of pharmaceuticals for therapeutic ends is drenched in dilemmas.

To explore these dilemmas, I will start in Chapter 2 by outlining the growth and dominance of pharmaceutical companies and of the medical profession who prescribe pharmaceuticals and I will note some of the trends that might constrain that growth and dominance. Chapter 3 details some dominant processes in relation to the expansion of pharmaceuticals, which can be labelled medicalisation, biomedicalisation and pharmaceuticalisation. Together these two chapters provide the foundation for building my arguments around pharmaceuticalised governance.

Chapters 4 to 6 build on that foundation to consider how pharmaceuticalised governance takes form in the everyday, the subjective and the interpersonal. The kinds of moral positions that are available to people in relation to the consumption or resistance to the consumption, of pharmaceuticals is discussed in Chapter 4. This chapter draws on research that attempts to provide insights into the consumption of pharmaceuticals and other medications in the household. Chapter 5 utilises this research to consider the decision-making practices in the home, noting the processes of self-diagnosis, experimentation and observation that occur. Chapter 6 further develops the argument by comparing home practices with those in other settings, particularly the general practitioner consultation.

Chapter 7 changes the focus to consider issues of governance at a population or public health level. Powerful public health concepts, such as herd immunity and the utilitarian underpinning of a population health approach that can be seen in vaccination policies, shape how we might think of other forms of medication practices targeted at an entire group or population. Chapters 8 to 10 continue to explore broader level issues, attending in particular to concerns about side effects, the conduct of clinical trials and the strategies that are used to promote pharmaceutical consumption. The importance of pharmacovigilance is highlighted, as well as the structural and interactional constraints that limit the success of pharmacovigilance endeavours. Chapter 11 then looks at different patterns and processes of pharmaceutical development and consumption in the Global North and the Global South indicating ways in which pharmaceuticals are entangled in processes of transformation of people, identities, professions and places.

Up to this point in the book there will be a sense of some very powerful social, political and economic forces that influence increasing levels of pharmaceutical consumption. Chapter 12 offers some reprieve from this vision, considering some important sites of resistance to processes of pharmaceuticalisation. Chapter 13 then pulls the arguments of the book together, but in a way that emphasises the complex processes of entanglement between pharmaceuticals and our lives.

## References

Albrow, M. (1970). *Bureaucracy*. London: Macmillan.

Billig, M. (1996). *Arguing and Thinking: A Rhetorical Approach to Social Psychology*. Cambridge: Cambridge University Press.

Blok, A. and Jensen, T. (2011). *Bruno Latour: Hybrid Thoughts in a Hybrid World*. London and New York: Routledge.

Bury, M. (1982). Chronic illness as biographical disruption. *Sociology of Health and Illness* 4 (2): 167–182.

Collin, J. (2016). On social plasticity: The transformative power of pharmaceuticals on health, nature and identity. *Sociology of Health and Illness* 38 (1): 73–89.

Costello, B. and Roberts, F. (2001). Medical recommendations as joint social practice. *Health Communication* 13 (3): 241–260.

Dew, K. (2012). *The Cult and Science of Public Health: A Sociological Investigation*. London and New York: Berghahn.

Fleck, L. (1979). *Genesis and Development of a Scientific Fact*. Chicago: University of Chicago Press.

Foucault, M. (1970). *The Order of Things: An Archaeology of the Human Sciences*. London: Tavistock.

Foucault, M. (1988). Technologies of the self. In: *Technologies of the Self: A Seminar with Michel Foucault* (eds L. Martin, H. Gutman and P. Hutton), 16–49. Amherst: University of Massachusetts Press.

Franklin, S. (2013). *Biological Relatives: IVF, Stem Cells and the Future of Kinship*. Durham and London: Duke University Press.

Gabe, J., Harley, K. and Calnan, M. (2015). Healthcare choice: Discourses, perceptions, experiences and practices. *Current Sociology* 63 (5): 623–635.

Harris, S. (2008). Constructionism in sociology. In: *Handbook of Social Constructionism* (eds J. Holstein and J. Gubrium), 231–247. New York: The Guildford Press.

Kuhn, T. (1970). *The Structure of Scientific Revolutions*. Chicago: University of Chicago Press.

Layder, D. (1998). From theory to data: Starting to theorize. In: *Sociological Practice* (ed. D. Layder), 100–132. London: Sage.

Parsons, T. (1958). Definitions of health and illness in the light of American values. In: *Patients, Physicians and Illness: Sourcebook in Behavioral Science and Medicine* (ed. E.G. Jaco), 165–187. Glencoe: The Free Press.

Pollard, S., Bansback, N. and Stirling, B. (2015). Physician attitudes toward shared decision making: A systematic review. *Patient Education and Counseling* 98: 1046–1057.

Porter, T. (1995). *Trust in Numbers: The Pursuit of Objectivity in Science and Public Life*. Princeton: Princeton University Press.

Scott, J.C. (1998). *Seeing Like a State: How Certain Schemes to Improve the Human Condition Have Failed.* New Haven and London: Yale University Press.

Steinberg, D. (2015). The bad patient: Estranged subjects of the cancer culture. *Body and Society* 21 (3): 115–143.

Williams, S., Martin, P. and Gabe, J. (2011). The pharmaceuticalisation of society? A framework analysis. *Sociology of Health and Illness* 33: 710–725.

# 2 The development of pharmaceutical hegemony

## The rise of the medical profession and its pharmacopeia

Common sites for the prescribing of medications are the primary care consultation room, general practice clinic and the hospital. In these spaces, medical professionals have the authority to determine whether a medication is prescribed, what sort of medication is prescribed and how long a medication should be taken for. A common sense view of this might assume that this situation was a natural outcome of the scientific expertise of medically trained personnel; they have the knowledge therefore they gained this right. But a common sense view is not the whole story. In this chapter, I will provide an account of the medical profession's rise to prominence, which suggests that other factors besides accurate knowledge of therapeutic interventions need to be taken into consideration to explain the contemporary situation of medical dominance.

There are great differences in the medical profession today from the medical occupations when they embarked on professionalisation strategies in the 1800s. In the 1800s physicians regarded themselves as a product of a liberal education, with medicine being a gentlemanly pursuit. As gentlemen, physicians were the elite of the medical profession mixing with other social elites (Nicholls 1988). Physicians diagnosed and prescribed, inhabiting the world of ideas and enlightenment thinking, but were above manual pursuits. As such physicians would not lower themselves to such things as making up medications. This was left to others, and in Anglophone countries these others were apothecaries. Apothecaries did not have the high status of physicians, particularly as their work was associated with trade (Nicholls 1988). That is, they were shopkeepers selling their merchandise of herbal preparations and other remedies.

It was not only the medical division of labour that has changed; therapeutic approaches have changed dramatically since medical regulation started to occur in the mid-nineteenth century. In the early part of the nineteenth century 'heroic medicine' had its heyday. Therapeutic approaches included a reliance on intensive general bloodletting carried out by venesection, and local bloodletting by the use of leeches. The label heroic derived from its intensive approaches, in contrast to more gentle approaches. Blistering was another treatment of choice, where a second-degree burn would be created, and would become infected and suppurate; the pus was seen as a sign of the infection being drawn out of the system (Kaufman 1971). Purging was carried out by the use of emetics, to induce vomiting and cathartics, to evacuate the bowels. Calomel (mercurous chloride) was also given in large doses for a variety of conditions. These massive doses produced salivation, loosening of the teeth, falling out of the hair and other symptoms of acute mercury poisoning. As calomel would irritate the bowel it was sometimes given with opium. These heroic measures were designed to restore the balance of humours in the body. Surgery was not a much better option with a surgical mortality rate nearing 20 per cent in some hospitals. The patient receiving surgery was likely to be drunk in order to numb the pain. The surgeon would have hands and instruments that were not sterile, and was likely to be wearing a frock '[s]tiff with dried blood of previous patients, the whole atmosphere fraught with pain and thick with bacteria' (Sigsworth 1972: 109).

This discussion about heroic medicine may leave us to wonder how people could submit themselves to such a toxic approach that seems like it was more likely to shorten lives than prolong them. But on the whole people willingly participated. Understandings of therapeutics meant that one should witness a physiological response to a medication – so salivating as a response to taking calomel could be interpreted as a wanted and expected reaction. Are our under-standings so different today? In the case of cancer, for example, highly toxic regimes are used for preventive and therapeutic purposes. Kirsten Bell (2010) found that cancer patients who were receiving chemotherapy would occasionally become distressed if they were not experiencing side effects from the toxic regime of treatment. This anxiety was an outcome of a belief that side effects would indicate that the treatment was working. But a major difference between heroic medicine and the medicine of today is the philosophical underscoring of the respective approaches. Heroic medicine was based on the theory of humours. The theory of humours was grounded on a view that the body needed to be main-tained in a state of good 'flow' to prevent blockage, and so evacuation of bodily fluids was a necessary part of maintaining health (Porter 2006). So for example, because it was believed that fever was caused by miasmas or noxious substances arising from filth and putrefying matter that corrupted the natural humours of the body, treatment for fever was aimed at driving out the vitiated humours (Duffy 1979). And this driving out could be quite drastic.

In the mid-nineteenth century medicinal practice started to take a very different shape, strongly influenced by the Paris Clinical School (Rosenberg 1987). Doctors came to see disease in quite a different way, in what Michel Foucault articulated as a shift from a medicine of health to a medicine of nor-mality (Foucault 2003). Instead of solely focusing on restoring the body to a non-diseased state, doctors now developed norms about the ideal physical state of the body. The concept of disease changed from one of a general physiological state to one where disease was the result of specific agents, in the body that could potentially be made visible. These agents included germs. Specific kinds of traces in the body were now increasingly associated with specific diseases, with hospitals, their laboratories and autopsies becoming important sites for the development of this new knowledge. Microscopes and chemical testing became key elements in diagnostic processes.

The role of the laboratory became an essential element in medical practice, first coming to prominence in Germany in the early twentieth century and having a major impact on reforms to medical education. With the development of laboratory tests that could identify the cause of infection or malignant tissue, and instruments being developed to gauge the activity of bodily organs, new possibilities opened up. One was the capacity to measure more accurately, and to compare measurements across time and across patient populations. With the accumulation of such measures, ideals of normality could develop, a process that fostered the standardisation of medical practices. I will revisit this issue of standardisation later in this chapter.

Before the invention of stethoscopes, electrocardiograms, laboratory diagnosis and the whole plethora of diagnostic instruments that exist today, patients and doctors would have available to them the same signs of the condition the patient was suffering from. Doctors would be led to their diagnosis by asking patients' questions, and looking at such physical signs as skin colour, the colour of the palate, and the colour, smell and even taste of urine. But with the invention of the stethoscope the doctor had available to him (or more rarely her) an instrument that delivered signs (sounds from the chest) that were not available to the patient. Now the doctor could diagnose on the basis of the unseen. From this point on, doctors could exercise more control over information than patients, and could decide whether to make information available to patients or not. It is during the nineteenth century that we see regulation that starts to limit the choices available to the patient, and the power of the patient declines as the medical profession comes to dominance.

The development of diagnostic and training approaches that we might recognise today had not developed when the medical profession became regulated and able to control who could be called a medical practitioner and in turn, who could have control over prescription medications. In the United Kingdom (UK) the Medical Act establishing the General Medical Council was passed into legislation in 1858 (in the United States [US] licensing laws took a lot longer to take effect than in the UK with apprenticeship systems being the common route to medical practice until the late 1800s).

Attaining the status of a regulated profession conferred great authority on the medical profession, allowing it to self-regulate as well as exert control over other health care occupations, such as nurses. Perhaps more importantly, the medical profession could 'set the very terms of thinking about problems which fall in their domain' (Dingwall 2008: 4). The health care occupations that came to form the medical profession, physicians, surgeons and apothecaries, were able to secure a monopoly over its scope of practice and secure high status through processes of political lobbying (Larkin 1983).

The 1858 UK Medical Act allowed the medical profession to exclude what we would now call complementary and alternative practitioners from the profession. Bonesetters, herbalists and others would not have access to the same status and privileges as medical professionals. In the UK, the one exception to this was homeopaths. At a time of heroic medicine what could perhaps be considered an opposing therapeutic approach, homeopathy, had a strong following, especially amongst the higher social classes. As a result of this support they were able to successfully manoeuvre to obtain a place within medicine. Medical homeopaths therefore found a particular place in the UK system, including having their own hospitals, which continue through to today. We will return to a discussion of homeopathy and other non-drug therapeutic approaches in Chapter 12.

With regulation the medical profession now had dominance over its own work. It was able to act in an autonomous way (Willis 1983). Andrew Abbott (1988) argues jurisdictional claims over work content have three parts: claims to classify a problem (diagnosis); claims to reason about it; and claims to take action on it (treatment). For the primary care physician or general practitioner in particular, the expanding use of pharmaceuticals into the twenty-first century provided the basis for the kind of work they do and the sort of treatment they provide.

## The development of the pharmaceutical industry

The increasing prestige of the medical profession through the mid-twentieth century is entwined with the development of a pharmaceutical industry and the capacity for modern drugs to alleviate symptoms, mitigate pain and fight infections. Over the twentieth century we witness a remarkable change in the way in which medications are prepared and evaluated.

In the nineteenth century, individual pharmacists compounded mixtures, made up decoctions, emulsions, tinctures, ointments, pills and many more preparations (Greene 2005). These preparations came from a wide range of materials with popular ingredients including aloes, pomegranate bark, castor oil, cocaine and mercury (Trease 1964).

The history of intellectual property and drug development takes some surprising twists. Antoine Lentacker (2016), in reviewing Joseph Gabriel's *Medical Monopoly*, notes an inversion in how patents were perceived. In the nineteenth century, the medical profession regarded the patenting of medicines, a process which at the time meant that the ingredients were kept secret, as unethical. Patents provided a monopoly to a drug company so that prices could be inflated. Ethical manufacturers renounced patents and marketed their drugs to medical professionals only. Patent medicine manufacturers marketed their drugs through the popular press. This situation led to the expansion of patented medicines with thousands of compounds on the market using branded names to hide the ingredients. The ground shifted, with the idea being promoted that patent medicines should have their chemical identities revealed, but a new drug formulation so patented would be granted exclusive rights to the manufacturer for divulging their trade secrets. Patented drugs now attracted particular symbolic value as having the protected status of being original (Lentacker 2016). Generic brands that followed, using the same formula, could be conceptualised as an inferior product.

The evolution of mass produced pharmaceuticals had its inception in nine-teenth century physiology and chemistry. In the first half of the nineteenth century, physiologists developed the techniques to isolate and purify drugs that were used as medicines, such as quinine from Peruvian bark and strychnine from the Indian tree *Strychnos nux-vomica* (Weatherall 2006), leading to the establish-ment of the experimental science of pharmacology. In 1899, aspirin was dis-covered, the most successful painkiller of all time (Hardy 2001).

The synthetic dye industry of the nineteenth century played a major role in the industrialisation of pharmaceutical production; the chemical skills developed there were applied to the development of new drugs (Weatherall 2006). Devel-opments in physiology led to other advances, like the discovery that myxo-edema, a condition caused by an underactive thyroid, could be treated by extracts of thyroid from sheep, and synthetic versions of this hormone were developed. Penicillin and other antibiotics appeared in the 1940s. War efforts too played a role in the development of industrial pharmaceuticals; technological changes allowing for the development of mass produced capsules and tablets occurred in the mid-nineteenth century, with the compression of tablets being modelled on the technology used to make bullets for firearms (Martin 2006a). Work to develop chemical warfare agents during the Second World War had positive therapeutic spinoffs with substances related to mustard gas found to be useful in the treatment of some cancers (Weatherall 2006).

Taking up drug-based solutions to problems can have a profound impact not only on patients but also on the medical profession and even our understandings of identity. The development of some drugs led to profound changes in the way in which the medical profession could present itself. Chlorpromazine, a drug used in the treatment of psychosis, was developed in the 1950s. Its effect on psy-chotic patients was dramatic, as was the take-up and use of the drug by psychia-trists (Dew *et al.* 2016; Martin 2006b). The capacity to pharmacologically control psychosis provided psychiatry with a credibility that had been challenged by sociologists and the anti-psychiatry movement. The new drug shifted percep-tions about this particular group of health professionals and how they worked, focusing clinical practice on a neurochemical view of mental disorders and providing less breathing space for psychoanalytic and other approaches to severe mental illness. This in turn impacted upon common or popular under-standings of mental illness and a new view of personhood. People's thoughts, feelings and perceptions could now be seen as mediated by neurochemical pro-cesses, and therefore potentially controlled or shaped by neurochemical inter-vention (Rose 2003).

With the technical capacities in place the scene was set for major pharmaceu-tical corporations to synthesise and test millions of compounds (Weatherall 2006) in attempts to make more profit in the health care market. The rise in sales of pharmaceuticals was rapid, rising in the US from US$300 million in 1939 to US$2.3 billion in 1959 (Greene 2005). The profit-driven agenda of the pharma-ceutical industry can be illustrated by noting that between 1975 and 1997, 1223 new pharmaceutical chemical entities were marketed but only 13 of those were specifically for treating tropical diseases afflicting those in underdeveloped countries (De Maio 2014; Lexchin 2006). Pharmaceutical companies focused instead on producing drugs for wealthier countries, in the process exacerbating increasing global inequalities, with research endeavours focused on benefitting those already in a better state of health. This is an illustration of what is known as the inverse care law, where those in least need get the most resources and those in most need get fewer resources (Tudor Hart 2000). The focus of drug companies on profit and the market, and limited regulation around drug development and advertising, has other unfortunate consequences, for example, the manifestation of drug tragedies.

## Thalidomide and drug regulation

In the late 1950s a drug called thalidomide was marketed as a sedative in many countries. The eventual identification of serious birth defects associated with the use of the drug played a role in attempts to regulate the testing and marketing of pharmaceuticals.

Prior to the twentieth century, medications were tested in an ad hoc manner with no accepted standard procedure. An early example of this is the development of the smallpox vaccine by Edward Jenner, who tested out his cowpox vaccine, made of pus taken from the cowpox blisters of milkmaids, by injecting the pus into the eight-year-old son of his gardener. He next injected the boy with matter from a smallpox lesion to see if the vaccine worked (Halliday 2007). If by luck the boy did not die then Jenner could claim success, and indeed he did go down in history as a hero of modern medicine.

Up until the twentieth century, medical preparations compounded by apothecaries or pharmacists were of uncertain therapeutic value. One reason for this was uncertainty around the potency of the medication; in terms of contemporary standards, the composition of any drugs used by medical practitioners in the nineteenth century was not standardised, therefore practitioners could only estimate the potency of the drugs they were giving. There were early attempts to provide some steer on the quality of drugs, such as the 1875 Sale of Food and Drugs Act in the UK. This act aimed to ensure that drugs contained the ingredients that were claimed and outlawed drug adulteration, but this Act did not regulate for the safety or efficacy of drugs (Abraham 2009).

In 1910, the idea of the biological assay, a test performed to measure the biological activity of a drug or remedy, was suggested by American authors writing in the *American Journal of Pharmacy*. Biological activity relates to the potential therapeutic effect of a remedy or its potency. At this time it was suggested that the biological potency of digitalis (from the leaves of the foxglove) could be assessed by a 'cat unit', that is, how many leaves it took to kill a cat (Porter 1995). The goal of standardising the potency of a medication set off a train of more complicated standardising processes. This was a result of having to standardise all instruments and procedures in tests so there could be more certainty that comparisons between tests were reliable. With the cat unit, it was found that different cats varied in their tolerance for drugs; a better unit needed to be found. Today most animals used in drug testing are bred for that purpose and in some cases, as with the OncoMouse, are genetically modified to enhance their research utility. Standardising went beyond the animals for testing. Further standardising impacted upon laboratory procedures, so that all laboratory workers followed the same methods.

An important element in the standardisation of medicine was the development and the use of statistical methods in medical research. In 1946, Austin Bradford Hill conducted the first randomised controlled trial (RCT), to assess the efficacy of streptomycin for the treatment of pulmonary tuberculosis (Porter 2006b). In a RCT, trial subjects are randomly assigned to either a treatment group who receive the intervention, or a control group who receive a placebo (Chapter 1 discussed the placebo effect). In addition, those who assess the treatment effects need to be 'blinded' as to whether a subject has received the treatment or not, to avoid the possibility that they may assess differently for those in the treatment group and the control group. This is known as the double-blind RCT. For a medication to be claimed as beneficial it must be shown, through this process, to work better than a placebo. A variation on this is that, instead of using a placebo, a new drug is compared to the standard treatment to see if it is more beneficial.

Nineteenth century medical men did not embrace the idea of using statistics as it challenged their views on the importance of clinical experience. Before statistics could get some purchase in the medical world, other concepts, such as the idea of the normal curve, had to become part of their way of thinking so that the 'normal' could be compared with the deviant (Hacking 1990). The word normal did not even appear until the mid-eighteenth century (Rose 2003). In terms of clinical trials, the deviant would refer to the positive deviation in outcomes that one hoped for from the use of a drug. So, in order to do something as seemingly simple as determine whether a drug is effective or not, a host of institutional and theoretical alignments had to occur. These complex formations, or assemblages as some might refer to them, permeate all aspects of medication practices. By the end of the twentieth century, RCTs had become the primary means of legitimating therapeutic interventions and were placed at the top of the Evidence-Based Medicine (EBM) hierarchy.

The role of the RCT in providing the evidence for the safety and efficacy of drugs gained impetus following the thalidomide tragedy. Thalidomide was first synthesised in 1954 and marketed as a sedative in many countries. The Food and Drug Administration (FDA), the organisation tasked with regulating drugs in the US since the 1930s, was not so quick to give thalidomide the green light. A medical officer of health given the application was not persuaded by the testimonials that were produced as evidence of safety and requested further information about the drug (Light 2010). Meanwhile reports of serious side effects of the drug in Australia, Germany and Japan started to appear, with over 10,000 babies born with serious birth defects after their mothers had taken the drug to treat morning sickness. Common visible defects included stunted arms and legs or the absence of limbs (Light 2010). As a result of the FDA's stalling action there were only 10 thalidomide babies born in the US (Timmermans and Berg 2003). The drug was withdrawn in the early 1960s.

As a personal reflection on this event, thalidomide was being prescribed at the time that I was born. From my early years I occasionally came across people my age who had no arms or missing digits, and these people were described to me as thalidomide babies. I knew of this as something of a medical tragedy, but only lately have I learnt of its significance in shaping how drugs are evaluated.

The thalidomide tragedy led to calls for more stringent means of ensuring drugs were safe. FDA regulations were tightened in the US with restrictions placed on how drug companies could advertise their products and new regulations on drug efficacy and safety placed the RCT as the gold standard in health care (Timmermans and Berg 2003). By the end of the twentieth century, RCTs has become a primary means of legitimating therapeutic interventions, placed at the top of the EBM hierarchy.

The pharmaceutical industry did not sit back in the face of increased regulatory requirements to simply allow the state to exert a hold over its activities. Soon after the FDA was granted increased powers to restrict advertisements and set standards for clinical trials, free market or neoliberal economists worked with the drug industry to promote deregulation (Nik-Khah 2014). One mechanism for this was the establishment of the Center for the Study of Drug Development (CSDD) in the US. The CSDD provided an 'independent' cover for drug companies producing studies that advanced drug company interests, and at the same time not allowing the data for these studies to be verified.

Neoliberals and the CSDD developed and promoted a number of arguments that continue to be used to foster deregulation, as noted by Edward Nik-Khah (2014). One such argument is that state regulation of drug companies keeps useful drugs from the market, for example, through 'drug lag', the delay caused by regulation during which clinically valuable drugs would not be on the market. The argument is made that a delay to market has consequences for patients who may miss out on the benefit of the drug, an issue that is particularly acute for those with life-threatening illnesses. Additionally, it is argued that regulation reduces innovation, and that advertising restrictions reduce the amount of information that consumers have, therefore disempowering them. Moreover, the CSDD suggested that clinical trials were an inappropriate way of assessing drugs, because they did not emulate how drugs are used when released to the market, instead the CSDD promoted naturalistic studies, which is the study of drugs once on the market. To only assess drugs when they are on the market would require rigorous pharmacovigilance processes, and this topic will be discussed in Chapter 10. In the early 2000s, the CSDD promoted the idea that the cost of bringing a drug to the market was a staggering US$800 million. This figure cannot be checked independently, as the data on which it was based on is confidential to the CSDD.

At a more abstract level, the CSDD put forward the argument that the state, through such agencies as the FDA, should not be the arbiter of science, a function given the title of pharmacologic Lysenkoism. This is a reference to a time in the Soviet Union when the adoption and enforcement by the state of the ideas of Lysenko, a biologist, were perceived to have had dire consequences for the Soviet people. Lysenko attempted to turn genetics into a Marxist science, dismissing some of the findings in western genetics as bourgeois. His ideas were enforced by the state, exacerbating famines that had featured in that country under Stalinism. The Lysenko Affair is celebrated by geneticists and molecular biologists as a prime example of why their activities should be self-regulating, and why the professional autonomy of science should be respected (Sapp 1990). This argument about the autonomy of science from the state was picked up by the CSDD.

The lobbying for reduced regulation of the drug industry has had some direct success in terms of drug approvals. In the 1980s, the FDA initiated expedited reviews to facilitate the rapid approval of drugs that could be used in the treatment of HIV (Saluja *et al.* 2016). The intention of these expedited reviews was that they would be used for life-threatening, untreatable or rare diseases, but drug companies now use this process for other drugs that are not exceptional (Saluja *et al.* 2016). In 1997, the FDA relaxed rules on advertising pharmaceuticals allowing for the development of direct-to-consumer advertising (DTCA), which will be discussed in Chapter 11.

The history of drug regulation since the thalidomide tragedy brings to the fore ongoing debates about the role of evidence in drug regulation and the influence of the state on the drug market.

### *Regulation of medical practitioners*

Along with attempts to regulate the pharmaceutical industry there have been many developments regulating the medical profession and placing limitations on the autonomy of the individual medical practitioner. Challenges to medical autonomy can come from empowered patients, and state support for other health professionals such as pharmacists and nurses to take on some of the tasks previously solely in the domain of medicine. This section focuses on another important challenge, the development and influence of the EBM movement, which became increasingly important in the 1990s. The goals of EBM include providing credibility to the medical profession by grounding therapeutic interventions in best science, and reducing the variation in clinical practice by developing evidence-based guidelines and recommendations. The evidence promoted by the movement is of a particular kind: clinical experience is downgraded in favour of findings from RCTs; and other forms of evidence of lower authority include the consensus of experts. Although the intention of the EBM movement was to base clinical decisions on the most appropriate evidence, which could include evidence from sources other than RCTs, RCTs dominate systematic reviews aimed at influencing treatment decision-making (Green 2000).

Since the 1980s, there have been a number of initiatives designed to ensure that practitioners remain competent after they have left the confines of medical school (Chamberlain 2013), and EBM has influenced the criteria used to assess competence. EBM recommendations are incorporated into codes of conduct and professional standards, including guidelines, protocols and practice policies. These are bureaucratic means of gaining conformity to EBM. Straying from guidelines and protocols can bring the practitioner to the attention of the medical profession itself, such as accreditation bodies and medical licensing agencies.

Oversight of medical practices additionally comes from those who manage institutions where medical professionals work, such as hospital managers, with management tools facilitating easier tracking of therapeutic interventions used by health professionals. The term 'scientific-bureaucratic medicine' has been used to depict this situation where bureaucracies oversee and control the implementation of evidence-based practice (Checkland *et al.* 2008; Lipman 2000). Through this management, medical practice can be more standardised, and defined as the logical and sequential application of science, undermining the clinical autonomy of practitioners.

Of course practitioners still retain a great deal of autonomy. There are many conditions for which guidelines are weak or have not been developed, and there are situations where practitioners may be able to justify taking a course of action that is not recommended in guidelines or dictated by protocols. A non-pharmaceutical example from my own research can illustrate this. In a study of the use of protocols in elective surgery, it was found that surgeons rarely used the protocols as designed. The protocols to prioritise who should access surgery were often in the form of a check list, with the intention that the surgeon would score on such things as the level of pain, the impact of social functioning and so on that the patient experienced. These scores would be added up, and if the patient got over a particular threshold they would be booked for surgery. However, when consultations between surgeons and patients were analysed, it was found that these protocols were not being used in this way; rather, the surgeons would determine whether they thought the patient should have surgery and subsequently fill out the protocols to align with their decision (Dew *et al.* 2005; Dew *et al.* 2010). Surgeons and other practitioners can base their rejection of protocols on the claimed importance of their clinical experience or acumen (Chamberlain 2013). Knowledge that is based in experience has been called indeterminate knowledge, which refers to claims that there are aspects of medical practice that cannot be codified or made technical (Jamous and Peloille 1970). There is too much uncertainty in medical practice, factors have to be weighed up and hunches based on past experiences followed up. Claims to clinical expertise can act as a form of resistance against external efforts to control the work of medical practitioners (Chamberlain 2013).

## Concluding comments

What I have tried to show here is that there are a number of historical developments that have interweaved to produce the contemporary situation where our main therapeutic approach relies on pharmaceuticals, many of which are prescription only and therefore, controlled by the medical profession. I have presented a case for a process of mutual shaping and interacting between the medical profession, the pharmaceutical industry and processes of standardisation and normalisation. It is not just the case that we, as a society, have developed a reliance, maybe we could call it a social addiction, to pharmaceuticals, but that the use of pharmaceuticals takes a particular form, embedded within the systems and institutions of our society. The requirement of drug companies to undertake RCTs, and the EBM movement placing RCTs at the top of their hierarchy of evidential authority, provide a powerful influence over clinical behaviour, intensifying the use of pharmaceuticals as the favoured therapeutic approach. Meanwhile, other therapeutic approaches are disfavoured, lacking the capacity to pass the hurdle of clinical trials. Any approach that requires manual skills or dexterity, or clinical expertise, has a more difficult time with clinical trials, because the treatment cannot be double-blinded. Any therapeutic approach that requires identifying the particular remedy for the particular person has a much more difficult time with clinical trials as you cannot simply divide a population into a treatment group and a placebo group. With RCTs dominating, pharmaceutical approaches gain the upper hand in gaining the credibility of the scientist.

The argument that the medical profession embarked on specific strategies to exclude competitors, and the kind of critique of how pharmaceuticals are developed and used that will be encountered throughout this book may, at times, read like a rather cynical and jaundiced view of medicine. There is another side to this, or a tension, that I think could be considered productive. There are explanations for why we embrace particular therapeutic regimes, at a broader cultural and social level as well as at a personal level. Today we may analyse and critique medical dominance, but in many instances we embrace it. We seek out people we can rely on, so that responsibility for decisions, particularly in situations that might be life-threatening, does not have to fall on us or at least on us alone. We have a lot to gain from the status quo. The desire to find a pill for every ill is a strong one, perhaps more so in societies where the productive worker is viewed as the central character in economic life, and economic life takes precedence over other issues. Personal health and economic health become entwined, and we are compelled to seek help from appropriate authorities. It is to these issues influencing our consumption of medications that we turn to in the following chapter.

## References

Abbott, A. (1988). *The System of Professions: An Essay on the Division of Expert Labor.* Chicago: University of Chicago Press.

Abraham, J. (2009). Partial progress: Governing the pharmaceutical industry and the NHS, 1948–2008. *Journal of Health Politics Policy and Law* 34 (6): 931–977.

Bell, K. (2010). Biomarkers, the molecular gaze and the transformation of cancer survivorship. *BioSocieties* 8 (2): 124–143.

Chamberlain, J.M. (2013). *The Sociology of Medical Regulation: An Introduction.* Dordrecht: Springer.

Checkland, K., Harrison, S., McDonald, R., Grant, S., Campbell, S. and Guthrie, B. (2008). Biomedicine, holism and general medical practice: Responses to the 2004 general practitioner contract. *Sociology of Health and Illness* 30 (5): 788–803.

De Maio, F. (2014). *Global Health Inequities: A Sociological Perspective.* Basingstoke: Palgrave Macmillan.

Dew, K., Cumming, J., McLeod, D., Morgan, S., McKinlay, E., Dowell, A. and Love, T. (2005). Explicit rationing of elective services: Implementing the New Zealand reforms. *Health Policy* 74 (1): 1–12.

Dew, K., Scott, A. and Kirkman, A. (2016). *Social, Political and Cultural Dimensions of Health.* Cham, Switzerland: Springer.

Dew, K., Stubbe, M., Macdonald, L., Dowell, A. and Plumridge, E. (2010). The (non)use of prioritisation protocols by surgeons. *Sociology of Health and Illness* 32 (4): 545–562.

Dingwall, R. (2008). *Essays on Professions.* Aldershot: Ashgate.

Duffy, J. (1979). *The Healers: A History of American Medicine.* Urbana: University of Illinois Press.

Foucault, M. (2003). *The Birth of the Clinic: An Archaeology of Medical Perception.* London and New York: Routledge.

Green, J. (2000). Epistemology, evidence and experience: Evidence based health care in the work of accident alliances. *Sociology of Health and Illness* 22 (4): 453–476.

Greene, J. (2005). Releasing the flood waters: Diuril and the reshaping of hypertension. *Bulletin of the History of Medicine* 79 (4): 749–794.

Halliday, S. (2007). *The Great Filth: The War against Disease in Victorian England.* Chalford, Stroud: Sutton Publishing.

Hardy, A. (2001). *Health and Medicine in Britain Since 1860.* Houndmills: Palgrave.

Jamous, H. and Peloille, B. (1970). Changes in the French university-hospital system. In: *Professions and Professionalization* (ed. J. Jackson), 111–152. Cambridge: Cambridge University Press.

Kaufman, M. (1971). *Homeopathy in America: The Rise and Fall of a Medical Heresy.* Baltimore: Johns Hopkins University Press.

Larkin, G. (1983). *Occupational Monopoly and Modern Medicine.* London: Tavistock Press.

Lentacker, A. (2016). The symbolic economy of drugs. *Social Studies of Science* 46 (1): 140–156.

Lexchin, J. (2006). The pharmaceutical industry and the pursuit of profit. In: *The Power of Pills: Social, Ethical and Legal Issues in Drug Development, Marketing and Pricing* (eds J.C. Cohen, P. Illingworth and U. Schüklemk), 11–24. London: Pluto Press.

Light, D. (2010). The Food and Drug Administration: Inadequate protection from serious risks. In: *The Risks of Prescription Drugs* (ed. D. Light), 40–68. New York: Columbia University Press.

Lipman, T. (2000). Power and influence in clinical effectiveness and evidence-based medicine. *Family Practice* 17 (6): 557–563.

Martin, E. (2006a). The pharmaceutical person. *BioSocieties* 1 (3): 273–287.

Martin, E. (2006b). Pharmaceutical virtue. *Culture, Medicine and Psychiatry* 30: 157–174.

Nicholls, P. (1988). *Homoeopathy and the Medical Profession.* London: Croom Helm.

Nik-Khah, E. (2014). Neoliberal pharmaceutical science and the Chicago School of Economics. *Social Studies of Science* 44 (4): 489–517.

Porter, R. (2006). What is disease? In: *The Cambridge History of Medicine* (ed. R. Porter), 71–102. Cambridge: Cambridge University Press.

Porter, T. (1995). *Trust in Numbers: The Pursuit of Objectivity in Science and Public Life*. Princeton: Princeton University Press.

Rose, N. (2003). The neurochemical self and its anomalies. In: *Risk and Morality* (eds R. Ericson and A. Doyle), 407–437. Toronto: University of Toronto Press.

Rosenberg, C. (1987). *The Care of Strangers: The Rise of the America's Hospital System*. New York: Basic Books.

Saluja, S., Woolhandler, S., Himmelstein, D., Bor, D. and McCormick, D. (2016). Unsafe drugs were prescribed more than one hundred million times in the United States before being recalled. *International Journal of Health Services* 44 (3): 523–530.

Sapp, J. (1990). *Where the Truth Lies: Franz Moewus and the Origins of Molecular Biology*. Cambridge: Cambridge University Press.

Sigsworth, E.M. (1972). Gateways to death? Medicine, hospitals and mortality, 1700–1850. In: *Science and Society 1600–1900* (ed. P. Mathias), 97–110. Cambridge: Cambridge University Press.

Timmermans, S. and Berg, M. (2003). *The Gold Standard: The Challenge of Evidence-Based Medicine and Standardization in Health Care*. Philadelphia: Temple University Press.

Trease, G. (1964). *Pharmacy in History*. London: Balliére, Tindall and Cox.

Tudor Hart, J. (2000). Commentary: Three decades of the Inverse Care Law. *British Medical Journal* 7226: 18–19.

Weatherall, M. (2006). Drug treatment and the rise of pharmacology. In: *The Cambridge History of Medicine* (ed. R. Porter), 211–237. Cambridge: Cambridge University Press.

Willis, E. (1983). *Medical Dominance: The Division of Labour in Australian Healthcare*. Sydney: George Allen and Unwin.

# 3    Expanding medicine

This chapter discusses sociologically informed understandings about the expansion of medicine, building on the description of the rise in status of the medical profession covered in the previous chapter. Medical dominance is not a term that is simply applied to the medical profession's occupational status in relation to other health care practitioners. It additionally applies to the way in which medical ideals and practices play an increasingly prominent role in all our lives. The term medicalisation has been used by sociologists to describe a process in which medicine increasingly dominates our lives under the oversight, or as a result of the influence of the medical profession. The medical profession is itself embedded within much wider social forces and networks, and some of these facilitate medicalising processes.

## Medicalisation

For many years I have taught a topic on medicalisation in a stage one university course in sociology. It is not uncommon for me to later cross paths with a former student who has taken that course years before. Although I lectured on many topics in that course, the topic of medicalisation is commonly the one that former students will spontaneously mention, sometimes suggesting that it was that topic in particular that got them excited about sociology, or it was that topic that allowed them to start thinking sociologically.

Medicalisation is a term that links up many ideas. It can be understood as a process whereby conditions that were once not treated medically come to be seen as medical problems, therefore coming within the domains of medical treatment and the medical profession. Medicalisation can be viewed in a negative light, as an almost cynical expansion of medical practices in order to further control particular populations. Furthermore, it can be seen as a way of avoiding confronting social issues by individualising problems. We can think here of something such as stress caused by intolerable workplace conditions. When the stressed person turns up at the physician's clinic, the diagnosis is not one of work-placed induced stress, requiring a reorganisation of the workplace, but maybe something like anxiety disorder caused by an overanxious person, which requires an anti-anxiolytic medication. The social problem has been individualised so that the status quo is protected, the cause of the problem is found in the individual and the solution is a medical one, which in this case may be drug-based.

Medicalisation can be seen in a positive light as well. Over recent times in New Zealand, as with many countries, there has been much debate about whether substance abuse and the use of recreational drugs should be considered as an issue of criminal justice or one of health. This debate has become particularly prominent due to concerns about a drug called 'P', or meth or methamphetamine. Using P is illegal and those caught with it are dealt with by the courts and may face prison sentences. But there is a strongly expressed view by many that the problem is a medical one. People become addicted to P and should not be punished, but treated. With successful treatment, P users might be able to avoid further criminalisation and take up a useful place in social life. The view of P as an addiction is a medically informed one. Addiction is a diagnostic category, which would make the condition one for doctors to deal with, rather than prison officers. There is an apparent struggle over whether to criminalise or medicalise the perceived problem.

These are not the only ways of perceiving the problem of P use; it can be seen as an issue of broader social trends, or what are sometimes called structural issues. For example, if we thought of people as using meth as a result of alienation from an unjust society, marginalisation in social life or a culturally facilitated desire for different forms of experience, our responses to the problem might be different, and might involve other agencies beyond penal and medical ones.

Viewing medicalisation as a trend, we might consider other behaviours that could be medicalised in the future. Currently there is a great deal of effort being put into reducing and even eliminating tobacco consumption and its negative health impacts. The use of vaping instead of smoking cigarettes may be promoted. Apps have been developed to help people who are trying to quit smoking, and the use of nicotine replacement products. In addition to these endeavours aimed at individual smokers, others include raising taxes on tobacco products and limiting sites of sale. If these trends continue, tobacco will start to become very expensive indeed, and increasingly difficult for poor people to purchase. For some this may help them quit, but for others the addiction to tobacco may prove a major problem. One solution to this would be to remove tobacco from general sales, whilst treating tobacco addiction as a medical issue. Those who are addicted could obtain tobacco products on prescription from a medical professional, moving the activity of tobacco smoking from the market place to the medical realm; tobacco smoking would be successfully medicalised. This may never happen of course, but it is the kind of development that is quite possible given the trend of medicalisation.

The term biomedicalisation has been coined to bring into focus particular developments influencing the shape and direction of medicalisation in contemporary times, since around 1985 (Clarke *et al.* 2010). The increasing role of information technologies is changing the way in which medical information is circulated and influences practices. Sarah Nettleton and colleagues suggest that biomedical conceptions of illness and cure dominate when people access the Internet for health-related issues (Nettleton *et al.* 2005). Features of biomedicalisation include the increasing surveillance through screening procedures and a concern with risk of future diseases, and with the idea of enhancing function. These will all be explored in more detail on 32–34. The Internet affords new marketing strategies for drug companies to target the consumer, allowing drug companies to become a new source of authority for patients. Furthermore, biomedicalisation emphasises the way in which identity can be shaped by diagnostic categories, as I will discuss in the case of the balding male towards the end of this chapter.

Gaining medical or social acceptance for extending the range of conditions that are suitable to be treated by pharmaceuticals enables the expansion of the medical market and the term 'pharmaceuticalisation' has been used more recently to capture this. Pharmaceuticalisation can be seen as both an extension of medicalisation in that it expands conditions that are treated medically, and a challenge to medical dominance in that medical professionals may not be in control of this expansion. Pharmaceuticalisation has been defined as the 'translation or transformation of human conditions, capabilities and capacities into opportunities for pharmaceutical intervention' (Williams *et al.* 2011: 711). The development of lifestyle drugs is an example of an opportunity being exploited by drug companies that target conditions that fall between medical and social conditions, such as hair loss and sexual potency. Other pharmaceuticals are marketed for a particular condition but used for lifestyle purposes, such as drugs for menorrhagia being used to delay menstruation during holidays (Fox and Ward 2008). Pharmaceuticalisation is a complex mix of biology, chemicals, expansion of disease classifications, consumer adoption and corporate interests.

There has been a great deal written on medicalisation, and the titles of some of the books dealing with the topic give a flavour of how it is approached. A few examples illustrate the focus these books have. An early example from Peter Conrad and Joseph Schneider (1992) is *Deviance and Medicalization: From Badness to Sickness*. This title emphasises the role that medicalisation plays in social control. The authors argue that there has been a shift from deviant behaviours being seen as immoral or sinful to those behaviours being given a medical meaning. They look at a number of examples including mental illness, alcoholism, opiate use and the medicalisation of childhood deviance. *Overdiagnosed: Making People Sick in the Pursuit of Health* by Gilbert Welch and colleagues (2011) provides us with the concept of overdiagnosis, and introduces its consequences: more sickness, more medical interventions, more side effects and adverse reactions. The focus on the act of diagnosis attends to the role of those doing the diagnosing, the medical profession, in fostering medicalisation. This book details the impact of screening for disease, and the ways in which that can lead to untoward outcomes, such as higher rates of unnecessary medical intervention. More on this later in this chapter. *Selling Sickness: How the World's Biggest Pharmaceutical Companies Are Turning Us into Patients* by Ray Moynihan and Alan Cassels (2005) focuses on the role of drug companies in medicalising processes and how they work to shape our perceptions of disease and drugs.

There are various ways that we can come to 'see' medicalisation at play. One commonly cited example is that of the use of amphetamines for the treatment of Attention Deficit Hyperactivity Disorder (ADHD). This is a contested disorder. Some people claim that the behaviours of children who appear out of control can be explained as a result of some chemical imbalance in the brain. If that is the case then correcting that balance, perhaps through pharmaceuticals, appears justified. For others, this explanation is seen as a way of controlling children and influencing parents and others to support this diagnosis and treatment, as the capacity of drugs such as methylphenidate to reduce the disruptive behaviours of children can support a number of interests. It may support the interests of schools as the diagnosis of ADHD in schoolchildren may mean that schools can obtain special resources and so schools may put pressure on parents to seek such diagnoses. Teachers may find life easier if a child is controlled by the drug, and of course the drug companies profit from such diagnoses (Baldwin 2000).

But how are we to adjudicate between these different claims? The prescribing rates of methylphenidate increased dramatically over a short period of time in the United Kingdom (UK), with a 15-fold increase in prescriptions between 1994 and 1997 (Baldwin 2000). In other parts of Europe, such as in France, use of the drug was rare. This suggests that an increasing medicalisation of children occurred over this time in the UK, but perhaps not in some other places. A counter argument to this may be that the children in France were undermedicalised. That is, more children in France could have benefitted from being diagnosed with ADHD and treated with amphetamines. It is not easy to determine in any definitive way what level of medicalisation is ideal. But with medicalisation comes side effects as pharmaceuticals are toxic substances (more of this in later chapters). Amphetamines certainly have a number of side effects, some of which can be severe and irreversible (Baldwin 2000). If that is of concern then one might prefer to risk under to over medicalisation.

State interests can also have a role in medicalisation. Vrecko discusses the pharmaceuticalisation of addiction, including the development of drugs to treat the 'craving brain' that can target a range of risky behaviours, such as the consumption of recreational drugs, overeating and gambling (Vrecko 2016). Anti-craving medications were not pushed through by drug companies, but rather became a focus of research after funding support was provided by the United States (US) government (Vrecko 2016). It was the state's interests in controlling the population, in this instance recreational drug users that, led to the development of these drugs. Michel Foucault's concept of biopower is useful for understanding these developments. For Foucault, biopower is evidenced in the way our personal health concerns become linked to state concerns and desires for a healthy and productive population (Rose and Miller 1992). The state increasingly attempts to regulate biological processes through interventions, with medicine being one important institution for instigating this regulation (Foucault 1988). The term biomedicalisation uses 'bio' in this sense of biopower, but also to refer to the importance of the biological sciences in biomedicine (Clarke *et al.* 2010). I will return to this important concept in Chapter 7.

There are many means by which medicalisation is promoted, including through the technology of screening and what has been called the molecularisation of medicine, and I will now turn to a discussion of these.

## Screening and pre-disease

Overdiagnosis was mentioned earlier. One important cause of overdiagnosis is the increasing practice of screening symptomless people for disease. The idea of checking healthy people for possible future health problems goes back to at least the mid-nineteenth century, and became commonly accepted practice in countries like the US by the 1950s (Raffle and Gray 2007). An early driver in recommending regular medical examinations came from insurance companies, in order to facilitate the setting of insurance premiums, an issue still with us today. Early screening procedures included the use of radiography for tuberculosis control, as well as screening for diabetes and cancer. Screening possibilities have since grown exponentially with developments in genetic testing.

So, how does screening relate to overdiagnosis? To take one example, there have been dramatic increases in the diagnosis of thyroid cancer, most likely due to the increased detection of subclinical cancers that would not, even without treatment, progress to disease. With this overdiagnosis many patients will receive treatment without any clinical benefit, and with a chance of having associated side effects from treatment (Davies 2016).

Some authors claim that there is a screening paradox, captured in the following quote:

> The greater the harm through overdiagnosis and overtreatment from screening, the more people there are who believe they owe their health, or even their life, to the [screening] programme.
>
> (Raffle and Gray 2007)

One reason for this paradox is what is known as lead time bias. To take the example of prostate screening, by introducing screening, cancer may be detected earlier, even before symptoms arise. The survival time for cancer is calculated from the point of diagnosis to a point of death. This gives the impression of increased survival from screening. Why so? I will try to explain this through a hypothetical example of two men, same age, with the same cancer at the same stage and progressing at the same rate. Bob undertakes screening and his cancer is identified at age 65. He lives for 10 years, so his cancer survival rate is calculated as a 10-year survival from the point of diagnosis. Jack does not undertake screening, but like Bob he develops some symptoms at age 70, and upon investigation, the cancer is diagnosed. He too lives to 75, but his cancer survival rate is calculated as a five-year survival from the point of diagnosis. So, although the outcomes are not at all different for the two men (with the possible exception of a longer period of anxiety and intervention for Bob), if we just considered survival rates we might think that screening has given Bob five years of extra life over Jack. Such distorted findings can encourage more screening, leading to more diagnoses and leading to more interventions. Those interventions can be invasive and reduce the quality of life for those with the earlier diagnosis. The originator of the PSA (prostate-specific antigen) screening test for prostate cancer shared this concern that the use of the test led to overdiagnosis (Bell 2010). This argument does not mean that all screening is bad. It just means that we need to think very carefully about when screening is appropriate.

Similar concerns can arise in relation to screening for the reoccurrence of disease. Clinical trial evidence on a biomarker for ovarian cancer, CA125, found that those treated when molecular signs of disease recurrence were detected fared no better than those treated when symptoms appeared (cited in Bell 2010). Treatment for ovarian cancer is likely to include the use of highly toxic chemicals that have unpleasant side effects. However, as noted in Chapter 2, patients may demand treatment with toxic substances for life-threatening illness even in the face of evidence to suggest it does not work. This treatment may be seen as inappropriate by some clinicians, but in the highly emotional situation of cancer, a treatment that does not work clinically may still benefit a patient's emotional well-being because something, rather than nothing, is being done.

Treating people to try to prevent or mitigate future risk of disease is a further expansion of medicalisation. The development of diseases of risk is informed by a population health perspective where risk factors for disease are identified, or thought to be identified. That is, a physiological factor is identified, which is regarded as indicating an increased risk for developing future disease. Actual disease does not have to be present, and may never occur, but the person is treated because of a calculation of future risk. Jeremy Greene suggests that we have seen a 'transformation from a symptom-bound to a numerically defined disease that could be conceived and treated according to the logic of risk' (Greene 2005: 793). Greene provides an in-depth study of the development of antihypertensive drugs in the 1950s, and other classic examples are high cholesterol levels for heart disease and high blood glucose levels for diabetes. If drugs can be identified, which change the person's physiology, such as reducing blood pressure or the level of cholesterol in the blood, then these diseases of risk can be pharmaceutically managed (Vrecko 2016). Illness is presented as something silent and unseen and markets for lifelong drug consumption are opened up (Dumit 2015). Diseases of risk create a new kind of patient whose physiology is a lifelong liability.

Chris Gillespie (2015) uses the term proto-illness to refer to the state people enter when risk of future disease has been identified through health screening procedures. Gillespie draws on elements of biomedicalisation, noting a shift in medical focus from symptoms of disease to the identification of biological signs of disease. These biological signs, or biomarkers, take on social meanings going beyond their biological meanings. Gillespie focuses on a number of features of the way identification of cholesterol markers as signs of future heart disease, and

PSA levels as signs of future prostate cancer, lead to new behaviours and relationships. Some of these changes in behaviour are forms of pharmaceuticalised governance. Gillespie refers to measured vulnerability, which we might see as a result of a PSA reading, to bring into sharp relief the way that statistical representations of future disease creates a sense of uncertainty for those identified as at risk, and influence how people live their lives (Gillespie 2015).

A proto-illness requires the newly identified at-risk person to take on new ways of acting, in some ways not dissimilar to the sick role discussed in Chapter 1. First, someone with proto-illness is required to increase medical contact so that, in Gillespie's examples, cholesterol and PSA levels can be monitored and interventions, such as the use of cholesterol-lowering drugs, can be adjusted. Second, everyday routines need to be restructured. In the event of those with proto-illness taking medications or supplements, for example, this might involve developing new routines around eating, as some medications and supplements must be taken at particular times in relation to food. Other general recommendations about lifestyle, such as exercise, were commonly made by health professionals when discussions about disease risk were had.

These changes to routine impact the proto-ill person's relationships, as other householders, friends and workmates might have to accommodate these requirements, or may be influenced in some other way by these changes. This is the third feature identified by Gillespie, a change in social relationships. Changed relationships include partners taking on the healthier lifestyle of the proto-ill; changes to contact with friends, as bars and parties may be avoided when alcohol is prohibited; and changes in relationships to work colleagues and bosses through, for example, the deliberate withholding of information about future disease risk, so as to avoid jeopardising future job prospects and access to health insurance (Gillespie 2015). Proto-illnesses foster particular forms of pharmaceuticalised governance, requiring changes in relationships with health professionals, friends, family and workmates and new routines that must be followed. The development of personalised medicine opens up more opportunities to identify proto-illness and to change the routines of those with actual disease.

## Personalised medicine

The development of molecular medicine facilitates the identification of disease markers, or possible future disease, much earlier, and to thereby institute earlier therapeutic or preventive interventions (Hogarth *et al.* 2012). Biomarkers play a central role in the extension of notions of proto-disease and physiological risk, and underpin the concept of personalised medicine as it is generally used. The much discussed development of personalised medicine promises a greater focus on 'the right person for the right drug'. It has the potential to change the nature of the surveillance of disease, monitoring of disease and diagnosis.

Personalised medicine has developed out of pharmacogenetics and efforts to predict drug reactions on the basis of genetic knowledge. Some terms related to personalised medicine include stratified medicine – the sorting of a population into biological groupings, for which particular therapeutic approaches can be taken – and precision medicine, where the people in particular groupings are closely monitored to identify changes in any disease markers in response to a tailored treatment (Day *et al.* 2017). The more extreme end of personalised medicine would see every person as a unique case requiring a specific approach (Prainsack 2018). Personalised approaches of this nature raise the possibility of selecting drugs that would lower the chances of adverse reactions occurring in the particular patient as a drug is selected for that person that fits best their risk to benefit profile. Personalised medicine raises a number of concerns including increasing expectations of success that may be unwarranted, further increasing inequalities in access to drugs as the cost of personalised medicine may make it inaccessible to the poor, and risks to the profitability of drug companies in a more segmented market as a result personalised drugs having a smaller market share (Williams *et al.* 2008).

An example of personalised medicine directed at biological groupings in patients is BiDil, the first drug approved by the US Food and Drug Administration (FDA) to be marketed for a racial group, African Americans (Pollock 2015). In clinical trials the heart medication was found to benefit black Americans. The mechanism of action of BiDil was not understood, that is, why it had a benefit for black Americans but no benefit for other Americans. Many commentators interpreted its marketing as an attempt to claim a biological basis for race, an idea that has been scientifically debunked. As Anne Pollock says, the physiological action of the molecule became entangled with the meaning given to that action (Pollock 2015).

Precision medicine is another associated term that refers to an increasingly precise action or effect of drugs. The precision of the drug is thought to lessen the chance of adverse reactions. Nikolas Rose refers to the neurochemical self when discussing the goal of drug developments that aim to affect only one neurotransmitter system, in the case of medications for mental illness (Rose 2003). Rose argues that the attention of psychiatry is now focused at the molecular level. The development of the drug Prozac was seen as heralding this new dawn of precision, molecular pharmaceuticalisation. There are moral consequences for such changes. Rose uses the example of alcoholism and the development of drugs to impact the desire to drink. As these drugs operate at the neurochemical level, hence Rose's reference to the neurochemical self, the alcoholic may no longer be considered deviant or aberrant, but as simply having disrupted neurochemical processes.

The excitement about the possibilities provided by precision medicine is captured by Sophie Day and her colleagues (2017) in their study of personalised medicine for breast cancer patients in the UK's National Health Service. Breast cancer patients are tested to identify a number of features that will determine what kind of chemotherapy they might be offered. For example, tests are used to determine if the cancer is oestrogen receptor positive, in which case they may be offered hormonal therapy, like Tamoxifen.

Perhaps better known to the public are the BRCA1 and BRCA2 genes that are deemed to increase the risk of cancer. Besides the use of prophylactic surgery, drug-based preventive measures can be taken, such as the use of Tamoxifen again (Bell 2010). Breast cancer patients are also assessed to determine if they have an amplification of the HER2 gene, which can be targeted by Herceptin (Day *et al.* 2017). One oncologist expressed the view that, through personalised approaches, cancer will be transformed from a frightening and aggressive illness to a chronic disease, much like diabetes. Such optimism about the possibility of targeted pharmaceuticals impacts not only staff in the hospital settings, but patients as well. Patients given a HER2 positive diagnosis felt relief, because it meant a specific drug could possibly help, even though the prognosis is not as good as for some other breast cancers (Day *et al.* 2017).

Day and colleagues (2017) suggest that what is referred to as cancer care personalised medicine can paradoxically lead to an increasing fragmentation of services, and move away from a more holistic approach that we might associate with the term personalised medicine. This fragmentation is an outcome of the increased monitoring of treatment effects that is required with the possibilities for adjusting medicine to better suit the recipient, aimed at improving the precision of treatment. Hence, the term 'precision' medicine might better capture the experience for patients of this form of medicine.

The development of biomarkers can provide leverage for patients in some circumstances in relation to accessing desired treatments. Kirsten Bell notes examples where patients were able to contest cancer specialists' seeming lack of concern about their anxieties by appealing to the evidence provided by biomarkers (Bell 2010). Patients could actively engage in treatment discussions rather than passively accept the opinion of their specialists.

Another outcome of developments in personalised medicine has been the availability of online genetic testing (Day *et al.* 2017), for example, 23andMe, an online genetic service that users pay to access. However, the information generated through using the service goes into a database, and can be sold on for a profit (Kragh-Furbo *et al.* 2017). This form of development can change our sense of self if we access this new information about our risk profile, which parallels the kind of changes that occur from any health screening. It also has consequences for others. If an individual discloses their genetic information to an online agency, they are disclosing information about those they have genetic connections to, that is, family. This allows the possibility for the companies, their researchers and their marketing agencies, who have access to the data, to make inferences about biological relatives (Prainsack 2018). What we might take to be our personal information is not just personal to us; it provides opportunities for others to target and influence those who are connected to us. Personalised medicine increases the power that biological information has over us, that is, it enhances what Foucault called biopower, and in the case of genetic information it has the potential to promote new forms of governance over broader groups of people by collecting individual examples of genetic information.

According to Rose, developments in personalised medicine and a focus on genetic and molecular medicine alters understandings of normality and pathology. He notes that with all the minor variations that have the potential to be found, everyone is now at future risk of some identifiable disease; as such, there is no longer any identifiable, stable state of normality (Rose 2009). The idea that there are molecular variations that could lead to physical or mental pathology, and which can potentially be corrected, means that the binaries of normal/ abnormal or normal/pathological no longer work. The breaking down of these binaries has had a long history, going back to what David Armstrong calls surveillance medicine.

A significant development in surveillance medicine was the Peckham experiment in England (Armstrong 1983). The experiment involved the establishment of the Pioneer Health Centre in a London suburb in 1935, open to local families, to assess the impact of preventive approaches to health care (Pearse and Crocker 1947). During the course of the experiment, it was determined that the 'treatable' population was much larger than expected. Of the first 500 families subjected to the health checks it was found that 32 per cent of family members had some disorder that was accompanied by disease, and another 59 per cent appeared to be well but had some underlying problem that should receive some sort of therapeutic intervention. Rather than focus on treatment of disease, health professions could shift their focus to its prevention, and a greater proportion of the population became subjected to health care interventions (Armstrong 1983). Today surveillance can be much more intense. Through genetic testing and other forms of identifying minor variations on our physiological responses, we are all on the pathological spectrum, and all of us might have the demands of self-monitoring and self-enhancement placed on us, as biological citizens required to support our lives through not only medications, but diet and exercise (Rose 2009).

A completely different way of thinking about personalised medicine is to consider the stance the state takes over the level of access to medications that citizens have. Some states heavily restrict the ability to purchase medications without the oversight of health professionals, and others leave it up to the market with very few restrictions (I will return to aspects of state regulation in later chapters). The state can loosen or tighten its grip on the drug trade, and I would suggest that we are more likely to see the state loosening regulations and so expanding the consumption of medications in the future. Sylvie Fainzang looks at the debates around and the impact of a French law of 30 June 2008 that opened up access to many medicines, which had previously only been accessible by prescription from health professionals (Fainzang 2017). This new law expanded the market for pharmaceutical consumption. For the state, this could ease its responsibility to cover pharmaceutical costs, as the purchases would be made through pharmacies and supermarkets without state subsidy. Additionally, the state promoted the idea that freeing up access to pharmaceuticals would provide citizens with greater autonomy and encourage citizens to be responsible (Fainzang 2017). This development perfectly illustrates Nikolas Rose's concept of responsibilisation. Rose refers to 'a double movement of autonomization and responsibilization' where 'politics is to be returned to citizens themselves, in the form of individual morality and community responsibility' (Rose 1999: 476). Fainzang suggests that the French state's promotion of self-medication practices fosters a personalised approach to therapeutics, where citizens are made responsible for working out what works best for them.

## Diagnostic inflation and changing thresholds

Diagnostic inflation is another means of enhancing medicalisation; it refers to the expansion of categories of diagnosable conditions. This process is easily observable in mental health. An influential factor in mental health diagnoses is the Diagnostic and Statistical Manual of Mental Disorders, shortened to the DSM. First published in 1952, the DSM is regarded by many health professionals as an authoritative guide for the diagnosis of mental illness (American Psychiatric Association 1952). Over the years there have been a number of iterations of the manual, and with each iteration there is an expansion of categories. In 1968, in DSM-II, there were 180 categories of mental disorder listed; by 1994 in the DSM-IV this had expanded to over 350 categories (American Psychiatric Association 1968, 1994).

The phenomenon of diagnostic inflation is where new categories of disease create new opportunities for drug companies. One commonly cited example of the creation of a new category is that of Social Anxiety Disorder (SAD), which appeared in the 1994 version of the DSM for the first time. The term social anxiety disorder provided pharmaceutical companies with an opportunity to market their products to combat this newly named condition. Paxil, a selective serotonin reuptake inhibitor (SSRI), was marketed to treat SAD, with marketing claims that it could be diagnosed in 20 per cent of the population.

Once a set of symptoms or signs has been accepted as pharmaceutically treatable by the health profession and patients, opportunities open up to expand the market for the drug used. A very easy way to instantly increase the potential market for a drug is to lower any thresholds or expand the criteria for who might use the drug. Greene notes the impact of trials undertaken in Veterans Administration Hospitals in the US on hypertension that formed the basis for recommendations to lower the threshold of diastolic pressure for antihypertension treatment. These clinical studies became a powerful marketing tool for the drug companies (Greene 2005). Gilbert Welch and colleagues (2011) in their book *Overdiagnosed* provide many other examples of this process. Dramatic changes occurred with the drug treatment of cholesterol. In the normal distribution of cholesterol levels in the American population, 200 mg/d is in the middle of the curve. Welch and colleagues note that over time the recommendation for anti-cholesterol treatment made by large health organisations in the US dropped from 300 mg/d, to 240 mg/d to 200 mg/d. Unsurprisingly, the drop to the mid-range of the distribution meant that 42 million Americans could now become targets for cholesterol-lowering drugs. Other examples with similar outcomes that they look at include drugs for diabetes and for osteoporosis.

Lynne Unruh and colleagues (2016) discuss the controversy over US guide-lines on who should receive statins to lower blood cholesterol. In 2013, the American College of Cardiology and the American Heart Association issued a new set of guidelines according to which nearly all men over the age of 60 should receive treatment. If these guidelines were to be used throughout the world, 1 billion more people would be targets for cholesterol-lowering drug treatment. The US guidelines were developed by professional associations; guidelines in some other jurisdictions are developed by governmental agencies, such as the National Institute of Health and Clinical Excellence in the UK. Research indicates that not only are guideline authors very likely to have finan-cial ties to pharmaceutical companies, including being paid as promotional speakers for the pharmaceutical companies and holding stock in the companies, but even voting members on the FDA's Center for Drug Evaluation and Research (CDER) have connections with pharmaceutical companies (Unruh *et al.* 2016). With such extensive conflicts of interest it must come as no surprise that recommendations for pharmaceutical intervention are being made to incorp-orate ever-widening sectors of the population.

## Medicalising baldness – an illustration

There are numerous examples that could be used to provide insight into the pro-cesses of medicalisation, biomedicalisation and pharmaceuticalisation. One study illustrating a number of these elements is from Kevin Harvey (2013), who researched how treatments for baldness are promoted online. I draw attention to this particular research because it nicely demonstrates, in some detail, the spe-cific strategies that are deployed on pharmaceutical company supported websites to promote the consumption of pharmaceuticals.

Harvey's study shows how commercial and market interests drive the process of medicalisation, placing pressure on medical professionals to conform to patient desires and demands in an era of patient-centred care. Since the last few decades of the twentieth century there has been at least a rhetorical shift in medical practice towards promoting patient-centred care and shared decision-making. In shared decision-making, the preferences and values of patients play an important part in any treatment plan (Reyna *et al.* 2015). Harvey's study indi-cates one way in which patient preferences and values may be shaped to align with the preferences and values of drug companies.

With the development of the Internet and drug company sponsored websites, greater opportunities have opened up for information about drugs, diseases and diagnoses to be targeted at health care 'consumers' and potential patients. Har-vey's analysis of websites targeted at men concerned about balding illustrates this development (Harvey 2013). Harvey notes a number of features of commer-cial hair loss websites. One important feature is the identification of a cause in what could be called a reductionist style (reducing cause down to one or a very few elements), and then clearly linking that cause to a medication that can combat it. Hair loss websites designate hair loss with the name androgenetic alopecia. This is a particular linguistic formulation that positions hair loss within the medical domain: it is a technical term, so it sounds medical. Androgenetic suggests something that is a result of DNA; so on first reading treating baldness may appear to be a hopeless fight against a genetic predisposition. But there is a solution. The cause is a male hormone, androgen, dihydrotestosterone (DHT), which affects hair follicles. An excess of this hormone, an outcome of genetic factors, causes hair loss. An available solution is to use drugs that counteract the effects of that hormone, one such drug being Propecia, which inhibits the conversion of testosterone into DHT.

The commercial hair loss websites position the balding man in a distinct way. Harvey notes the strategies used to depict the balding man as someone who has a spoiled identity. Spoiled identity is a concept famously developed by Erving Goffman. One can attain a spoiled identity through having visible bodily blemishes, or what Goffman dramatically refers to as bodily abominations (Goffman 1963). The hair loss websites depict hair loss as a blemish, one that can be fixed with drugs. One way of constructing the balding man as stigmatised is through visual depictions. Harvey notes that images used of the balding man are passive, in which the balding man is not engaged with the viewer – they may be looking in the distance, isolated from others. In contrast, the hirsute man, who has saved his hair through the use of drugs, is engaged with the viewer – usually looking straight at the viewer and beaming a smile. The balding man is therefore, cast as a particular type of man, one who is separated out from others and who does not have the enjoyment of life that others have. These men are constructed as less attractive, less assertive and less successful. Such representations are designed to induce anxiety so that a solution needs to be obtained – a pharmaceutical solution.

A final feature to mention is the suggestion by these websites that viewers use the information they have gleaned to facilitate a discussion with their health practitioners, who are able to prescribe the remedy. Websites use self-diagnosis tools so that potential pharmaceutical consumers can see what they have to do to combat balding. Websites often have some sort of quiz or checklist, which claim to predict your future. Harvey's own hair loss diagnostic report informed him that he had a '97.8% chance' of losing his hair by the time he was 49 (Harvey 2013: 707). Mary Ebeling notes that checklists for self-diagnosis on branded drug websites always provide a doctor discussion guide for prospective patients to use when they consult their physician (Ebeling 2011). In some cases, input from the website user can be used to fill a printable physician's report that the patient can take to their doctor. Pharmaceutical companies so deploy patients to persuade doctors and so the companies 'seek to dictate the course of the consultation by proxy' (Harvey 2013: 708). Here we clearly see that medicalisation is expanded out beyond the activities of the medical profession and incorporates drug companies and patients themselves. The incorporation of these other actors may challenge or undermine medical dominance, under the guise of patient-centred medicine.

## Enhancing life

Propecia is an example of trying to stave off, through pharmaceuticals, what might be considered normal biological processes. There is of course variation in how people respond to this. Some may consider the use of drugs to enhance our biological processes as positive. Drugs can be used to alter biological processes to enhance our experiences and comfort, or to enhance our chances of being more productive in the workplace and other environments. Contraceptives have been used to suppress menstruation, and not only has this been viewed as having lifestyle appeal for some women, but it is seen as the appropriate thing to do for women in some environments, such as deployed military personnel (Collin 2016). The expansion of the use of drugs so that people can function better in particular work situations is one that may gain further purchase. In some work-places, pharmaceutical use has been obligatory for some time, for example, the requirement for medical personnel to have various vaccines, such as the yearly 'flu shot'. In relation to over-the-counter medications, the advertising claims about energising life compels citizens 'to exercise moral responsibility for themselves by purchasing such readily available products' (Hodgetts *et al.* 2017).

The development of drugs to maintain or enhance sexual performance in ageing bodies has been popularly embraced. For men, this has been evident for some years with the success of drugs like Viagra, which was approved by the FDA in 1998. For women, developments have been more recent with drug companies successfully lobbying for a condition of female hypoactive desire disorder to be recognised so that a potential treatment for this condition, a drug called Flibanserin, could be marketed. Flibanserin was approved in 2015. The development of drugs to enhance sexual performance are, according to Barbara Marshall, revising standards of sexual functioning, with active sexuality becoming a marker of successful ageing (Marshall 2010).

The process of using medications to enhance performance also occurs in the area of emotions and affect. Emily Martin (Martin 2006) interviewed a pharmaceutical marketer who stated that psychiatrists combined different drugs into cocktails for their patients for this purpose. One example is known as the Hollywood Cocktail: the combination of psychoactive drugs is given to sedate the patient, but in addition activate them and give pep, so that the patient is not simply restored to a normal state, but is better than normal and in a state of hyper-alertness (Martin 2006). So-called smart drugs, used as cognitive enhancers, such as Methylphenidate and Modafinil, have been used by university students to enhance performance, linking the use of these drugs to a competitive ethic in student education (Collin 2016).

Drugs to enhance our normal capacities, instead of restoring us to normality, are likely to increasingly appeal to many groups in society, particularly if drugs are able to give people a competitive edge. The most visible social situation where this is a constant occurrence, but one troubling for sports bodies, is on the sports field.

## Concluding comments

At the time of writing this, the last time I saw my general practitioner he asked me how I felt about taking a blood test to assess my cholesterol levels. He presented this inquiry in quite a tentative manner, possibly because he did not really think I needed a test, or because he felt this was something he had to do rather than something he wanted to do. I responded by saying something along the lines that I realised this was something he had to do to align with clinical guidelines, and I knew that there were funding implications for his practice if I did not agree to the test, so I would go along with his suggestion. This little incident reveals a great deal about current forces of medicalisation and their policy, interactional and clinical embeddedness.

Cholesterol testing and other physiological tests are increasingly built into protocols and guidelines for medical practitioners so that they are expected to offer blood tests to their patients. Expectation can turn into a very powerful incentive if such testing is tied to funding, or to an assessment of the adequacy of the clinician's practice. This can be done through the development of such technologies as performance indicators for health practices. Performance indicators can be tied to financial reimbursement for those health practices, or can be tied to quality assurance assessments and medical recertification. So, for example, a performance indicator might be that 80 per cent of the over 50-year-old patients of an enrolled practice need to be tested for cholesterol, and if this target is not met that practice will have state funding withheld.

This process of medicalisation links up a very complex set of ideas and practices: the concept of diseases of risk needs to be embedded in clinical practice, screening technologies need to be developed to assess the physiological process, panels of experts need to be persuaded to lower thresholds for risk, governing agencies need to be persuaded that the drugs will promote a healthy population and perhaps lower health costs over the long term, facilities need to be developed to monitor the performance of medical practitioners, rules or guidelines need to be put in place to assess what is appropriate for those practitioners to do, and the patient population needs to be persuaded that all of this is in its best interests. What a fascinatingly intricate interplay of actors, technologies and biologies is seen in the dance of medicalisation.

Medicalisation and pharmaceuticalisation are not simply one way processes. Chapter 12 will revisit this topic in exploring some of the forms and processes of resistance to pharmaceuticalisation, but the view that our lives are becoming increasingly medicalised and pharmaceuticalised is a compelling one. The next three chapters shift focus on to an exploration of how people in their everyday lives respond to these trends in medicalisation and pharmaceuticalisation.

# References

American Psychiatric Association. (1952). *Diagnostic and Statistical Manual of Mental Disorders.* Washington, DC: American Psychiatric Association.

American Psychiatric Association. (1968). *Diagnostic and Statistical Manual of Mental Disorders, Second Edition: DSM-II.* Washington, DC: American Psychiatric Association.

American Psychiatric Association. (1994). *Diagnostic and Statistical Manual of Mental Disorders, Fourth Edition: DSM-IV.* Washington, DC: American Psychiatric Association.

Armstrong, D. (1983). *Political Anatomy of the Body: Medical Knowledge in Britain in the Twentieth Century.* Cambridge: Cambridge University Press.

Baldwin, S. (2000). Living in Britain: Why are so many amphetamines prescribed to infants, children and teenagers in the UK? *Critical Public Health* 10 (4): 453–462.

Bell, K. (2010). Biomarkers, the molecular gaze and the transformation of cancer survivorship. *BioSocieties* 8 (2): 124–143.

Clarke, A., Shim, J., Mamo, L., Fosket, J.R. and Fishman, J. (2010). Biomedicalization: A theoretical and substantive introduction. In: *Biomedicalization: Technoscience, Health and Illness in the U.S.* (eds A. Clarke, L. Mamo, J.R. Fosket, J. Fishman and J. Shim), 1–44. Durham and London: Duke.

Collin, J. (2016). On social plasticity: The transformative power of pharmaceuticals on health, nature and identity. *Sociology of Health and Illness* 38 (1): 73–89.

Conrad, P. and Schneider, J. (1992). *Deviance and Medicalization: From Badness to Sickness.* Philadelphia: Temple University Press.

Davies, L. (2016). Overdiagnosis of thyroid cancer. *British Medical Journal* 355: i6312.

Day, S., Coombes, R.C., McGrath-Lone, L., Schoenborn, C. and Ward, H. (2017). Stratified, precision or personalised medicine? Cancer services in the 'real world' of a London hospital. *Sociology of Health and Illness* 39 (1): 143–158.

Dumit, J. (2015). Pharmaceutical witnessing: Drugs for life in an era of direct-to-consumer advertising. In: *The Pharmaceutical Studies Reader* (eds S. Sismondo and J. Greene), 33–47. Chichester: John Wiley & Sons.

Ebeling, M. (2011). 'Get with the program!': Pharmaceutical marketing, symptom checklists and self-diagnosis. *Social Science and Medicine* 73: 825–832.

Fainzang, S. (2017). *Self-Medication and Society: Mirages of Autonomy.* Abingdon: Routledge.

Foucault, M. (1988). The political technology of individuals. In: *Technologies of the Self: A Seminar with Michel Foucault* (eds L. Martin, H. Gutman and P.H. Hutton). Amherst: University of Massachusetts Press.

Fox, N.J. and Ward, K.J. (2008). Pharma in the bedroom … and the kitchen. … The pharmaceuticalisation of daily life. *Sociology of Health and Illness* 30 (6): 856–868.

Gillespie, C. (2015). The risk experience: The social effects of health screening and the emergence of proto-illness. *Sociology of Health and Illness* 37 (7): 973–987.

Goffman, E. (1963). *Stigma: Notes on the Management of Spoiled Identity.* Englewood Cliffs: Prentice-Hall.

Greene, J. (2005). Releasing the flood waters: Diuril and the reshaping of hypertension. *Bulletin of the History of Medicine* 79 (4): 749–794.

Harvey, K. (2013). Medicalisation, pharmaceutical promotion and the Internet: A critical multimodal discourse analysis of hair loss websites. *Social Semiotics* 23 (5): 691–714.

Hodgetts, D., Young-Hauser, A., Chamberlain, K., Gabe, J., Dew, K. and Norris, P. (2017), Pharmaceuticalisation in the city, *Urban Studies* 54 (15): 3542–3559.

Hogarth, S., Hopkins, M. and Rodriguez, V. (2012). A molecular monopoly? HPV testing, the Pap smear and the molecularisation of cervical cancer screening in the USA. *Sociology of Health and Illness* 34 (2): 234–250.

Kragh-Furbo, M., Wilkinson, J., Mort, M., Roberts, C. and MacKenzie, A. (2017). Biosensing networks: Sense making in consumer genomics and ovulation tracking. In: *Quantified Lives and Vital Data: Exploring Health and Technology Through Personal Medical Devices* (eds R. Lynch and C. Farrington), 47–69. Basingstoke: Palgrave.

Marshall, B.L. (2010). Science, medicine and virility surveillance: 'Sexy seniors' in the pharmaceutical imagination. *Sociology of Health and Illness* 32 (2): 211–224.

Martin, E. (2006). The pharmaceutical person. *BioSocieties* 1 (3): 273–287.

Moynihan, R. and Cassels, A. (2005). *Selling Sickness: How the World's Biggest Pharmaceutical Companies Are Turnings Us into Patients.* New York: Nation books.

Nettleton, S., Burrows, R. and O'Malley, L. (2005). The mundane realities of the everyday lay use of the Internet for health, and their consequences for media convergence. *Sociology of Health and Illness* 27 (7): 972–992.

Pearse, I.H. and Crocker, L.H. (1947). *The Peckham Experiment: A Study in the Living Structure of Society.* London: George Allen and Unwin.

Pollock, A. (2015). BiDil: Medicating the intersection of race and heart failure. In: *The Pharmaceutical Studies Reader* (eds S. Sismondo and J. Greene), 87–105. Chichester: Wiley Blackwell.

Prainsack, B. (2018). The 'we' in the 'me': Solidarity and health care in the era of personalized medicine. *Science, Technology and Human Values* 43 (1): 21–44.

Raffle, A. and Gray, J.A.M. (2007). *Screening: Evidence and Practice.* Oxford: Oxford University Press.

Reyna, V., Nelson, W., Han, P. and Pignone, M. (2015). Decision making and cancer. *American Psychologist* 70 (2): 105–118.

Rose, N. (1999). Inventiveness in politics. *Economy and Society* 28 (3): 467–493.

Rose, N. (2003). The neurochemical self and its anomalies. In: *Risk and Morality* (eds R. Ericson and A. Doyle), 407–437. Toronto: University of Toronto Press.

Rose, N. (2009). Normality and pathology in a biomedical age. *Sociological Review* 57 (2 suppl): 66–83.

Rose, N. and Miller, P. (1992). Political power beyond the state: Problematics of government. *British Journal of Sociology* 43 (2): 173–205.

Unruh, L., Rice, T., Vaillancourt Rosenau, P. and Barnes, A. (2016). The 2013 cholesterol guideline controversy: Would better evidence prevent pharmaceuticalization? *Health Policy* 120: 797–808.

Vrecko, S. (2016). Risky bodies, drugs and biopolitics: On the pharmaceutical governance of addiction and other 'diseases of risk'. *Body and Society* 22 (3): 54–76.

Welch, H.G., Schwartz, L. and Woloshin, S. (2011). *Overdiagnosed: Making People Sick in the Pursuit of Health.* Boston: Beacon Press.

Williams, S., Martin, P. and Gabe, J. (2011). The pharmaceuticalisation of society? A framework analysis. *Sociology of Health and Illness* 33: 710–725.

Williams, S.J., Gabe, J. and Davis, P. (2008). The sociology of pharmaceuticals: Progress and prospects. *Sociology of Health and Illness* 30 (6): 813–824.

# 4 Moral forces and medicine

## Introduction

In the last chapter, the expansion of medicine and some of its advantages and disadvantages was discussed. We might take the position that some of the influences on pharmaceuticalisation, particularly those coming from some of the drug companies, are immoral, because it puts profit before the health of those who consume the drugs. There are moral issues facing individuals seeking out therapeutic help. At a very basic level, moral issues can be seen in your response to a medical recommendation. Do you follow it or not? You are making a choice and therefore you are deciding on the right thing to do. In this chapter, the focus is on the moral positioning that individuals take when they make decisions about treatment options that require the consumption of pharmaceuticals.

When we are talking about morals we are talking about what we see as good and what we see as bad. We conduct ourselves, or act in the world, in relation to our morals. Morality acts as a disciplining mechanism as we pursue an ideal of being a good person. We may see ourselves as good or bad because we take medicine, or because we avoid medicines, or we might see medicines themselves as simply good or bad. What is important to note here is that the moral position we take on medicines shapes our behaviours and social practices in many ways. Medicines play a role in governing us.

My own understandings of the moral issues at play in the consumption of medicines go back a long way, but the issue of morality became most sharply drawn in relation to vaccines. This chapter does not focus on vaccines, there is much more on this in Chapter 7, but I will just touch upon some of these moral concerns here to indicate the sort of issues we might confront when taking medications.

In Chapter 7, I note my early research into vaccine-related issues and the ethical dilemmas they can create. During this research, I had contact with an organisation in New Zealand called the Immunisation Awareness Society (IAS). This organisation had a motto of promoting informed choice in relation to vaccinations, and gathered together information that challenged the position on vaccinations taken by medical and health policy institutions. When I was in contact with this organisation, they asked me if I would help out at an information desk during a health expo in Wellington, and I said I would do so for an hour. I turned up for my stint standing at a table and responding to the odd inquiry about what the IAS was all about. At one point I was confronted by a woman who was very angry for what I was doing. She was very concerned that we were getting people to think about vaccines for their children, rather than people simply following the recommended guidelines. Her concern was that if people thought about it some might make the wrong decision and not have their children vaccinated. This kind of argument, at that time, was not a problem to me, as I wanted to foster more reflective processes of medication consumption, so if people chose not to vaccinate after being better-informed that was their choice. If they chose to vaccinate after being better-informed, that was also their choice. I was simply advocating a position where people who wanted to, could know a little more about the issues before making a decision.

During my conversation with this woman, she took a very strong moral position that what I was doing was dangerous, with suggestions that it was evil. There was a reason for taking that position. She divulged that her child had a condition, which meant that she was very vulnerable to infectious diseases. Even more difficult for this mother was that she had been advised not to give her child vaccines because of her child's compromised immune system. For this woman, a mother of a very immune-compromised child, it was imperative for her child's safety that vaccines worked and that herd immunity was achieved so that infectious diseases did not circulate through the community. My simple desire to promote an informed public was, for her, a threat to her child's life. This is a dramatic example of the stakes that can be at play when it comes to the consumption of medicines and vaccines, illustrating that different value positions can clash dramatically. However, this chapter does not focus on the dramatic but on the more subtle understandings that people bring to medication use.

In addition to confronting moral issues in real life, there are many sociological influences that shape my interest in morals and medications. These are in no specific order but the first I will mention is Émile Durkheim, the first person to have the title of Professor of Sociology. Durkheim's work was underpinned by the idea that there are contradictory moral forces at play in society that influence individuals and collectives, most famously seen in his concepts of anomie, egoism, altruism and fatalism (Taylor and Ashworth 1987). From this perspective, moral forces are manifest in our social interactions and practices. Another potent influence is the work of Michel Foucault, who put a great deal of his scholarly energy into exploring the kinds of influences that shape our behaviours and practices, captured particularly forcefully in his concept of governmentality, noted in Chapter 1. Governmentality can be defined as the governing of the self and the governing of others through everyday activities (Lemke 2001). In the case at hand, governing occurs through the everyday practice of medication use. The final influence I will mention comes out of an approach to analysing text and talk called discourse analysis. In early sociological work using discourse analysis, Nigel Gilbert and Michael Mulkay (1984) developed the concept of interpretive repertoires. Interpretive repertoires are used by people (scientists in their particular study) to justify the understandings that they are conveying in their talk, but more than this, to achieve some sort of action through their talk. Applying the notion of repertoires here, one thing that is achieved when people talk about medication use is a moral position in relation to pharmaceuticals. These rather abstract ideas will become clearer as this chapter unfolds.

Finally, my understanding of pharmaceuticalised governance was an outcome of analysing and interpreting data on householders' understandings of medications and from being asked to write for a special issue of the journal *Social Science and Medicine*. The special issue was on pharmaceuticalisation. In writing up an article for this special issue, where our research team focused on the moral underpinnings of medication consumption, it became apparent that not only did this relate to the concept of pharmaceuticalisation, but that we could perhaps advance a particular and, at least for us, insightful understanding of that very concept through hybridising it with Foucault's concept of governmentality. These different influences facilitated me in developing the concept of pharmaceuticalised governance, where moral forces entwine with medication use and aspects of our conduct are governed through the routine use of pharmaceuticals, or resistance to their use (Dew *et al.* 2015).

## Generating stories

The material that I will use to illustrate possible moral positions in relation to medication practices is drawn from research that was undertaken by a team that included social psychologists, a social pharmacist and a number of PhD students and Master's students. I got involved in this research when Kerry Chamberlain, a critical social psychologist whom I knew of, but did not really know at the time, rang me and asked me if I would be interested in joining a team he was trying to put together to explore how people used medications in the home. Before Kerry told me about the project I geared up pretty quickly to say 'thanks but no thanks' to any offer of more research as I felt that my research plate was very full at the time. However, as soon as he started to tell me about his ideas, I thought this could be very intriguing. I was not aware of much research around that looked at how families and other households negotiated the use of medications in homes. I had no idea what we might find, and so the research was of interest to me. I did know that such an exploration would very likely identify all sorts of tensions as, since my wife and I now had a family with two boys, we had a whole set of different responsibilities in relation to medication practices, and we were often negotiating those practices. Should we take them to the doctor to deal with their ailments, or to an alternative practitioner, or should we just leave it to the powers of nature and time to bring about healing? Who would oversee any medication regimes that were recommended? How would we judge when to try something else, or stop giving a medication to one of our boys and so on and so on? These questions hooked me in and I began wondering how other households negotiate such things and what else was going on of which I was not aware.

As a research team we made an early decision that all of us would be involved in the collection of data, and our research design was quite complex. It involved getting all householders to agree to participate in the research, then if possible meeting them all in their home. At the first meeting, a map was drawn of the house and participants identified where medications were kept. We kept the definition of medications as broad as possible, referring to anything people took specifically for therapeutic value or as a preventive. We then asked participants to bring out all the medications in the house (at least all they were happy to bring out), to be placed on a kitchen table, coffee table or on the floor. Subsequently we did what could be called a medication-elicitation interview. We went through each medication asking what it was for, how it got into the home, who suggested taking it and where it was obtained. This was a truly fascinating process for many reasons. Medicines often evoked complex and detailed stories. As participants picked up a medication and looked at the bottle, they would start to recall who the medication was for and when it was first taken with stories that might take them to different locations around the world, different times and across generations. The act of picking up the material object seemed to generate spontaneous and unrehearsed stories, stories that were often being developed in the moment. Another fascinating element, discussed in this chapter, was the moral evaluations that people provided in relation to medication consumption.

That was not the end of data collection. We then asked one householder to take photographs over a period of a week of anything that they wanted to that was related to medicines. We asked another householder to keep a diary of all the medications taken in the household over the period of a week. Finally, we got someone else to keep a diary to record reflections on medications that they had over one week, and asked them to think about one issue at the end of the day. After two or more weeks we went back to interview the participants, using the diaries and photographs to elicit more stories. In the following I outline four different moral perspectives in relation to medication practices that we discerned in this research.

## Moral positions

In thinking about the information we had collected in relation to repertoires, we came up with four overarching positions that householders took in relation to their medication, which we related to different ideas about order (Dew *et al.* 2015). We labelled the repertoires as a restoring order repertoire, a disordering substances repertoire, a disordering body repertoire and a disordering society repertoire.

The restoring order narrative is one that we might expect, as it explains why we seek out medications in the first place and what we hope to achieve through their consumption. Pharmaceuticals can sustain or restore order, and many householders described medications using metaphors of balance, like keeping on an even keel. This restorative function was referred to even in the absence of 'evidence' of benefits from taking medications. Following a prescribed medication regime can signify obedience and conformity to what is a taken-for-granted good provided by a pharmaceutical industry that attempts to develop therapeutic agents to help us. Pharmaceuticals can signify trust in expert health providers. They can even have a talismanic quality of warding off illness. At one level, using this repertoire can justify not having to take responsibility for decision-making about pharmaceuticals, as trusted experts can make the decisions for you. In this repertoire there is a duty to be a responsible consumer or patient. Some householders took a more active role in making positive decisions to use pharmaceuticals because they do help them function, particularly in the face of chronic health conditions where order might not be able to be completely restored.

The restoration of order can come with a price but one that the user is happy to pay. For Lisa it is 'important to me to keep on taking the Lithium' despite it having an effect on her blood pressure and thyroid, which was 'a wee titch out of kilter'. Lisa downplays potential problems of the medication as a 'wee titch' because she 'would be really terrified of not taking' Lithium. When her partner, Bruce, was asked about what he took in relation to the medications that had been brought out from their storage places he said 'shit loads here':

> Cholesterol pills … gout tablet. … These are for my diabetes … this is something for blood pressure, I think…. These ones look after my liver…. I don't know what they do but I have some of them every day anyway…. I just do what the man says.

Bruce takes a great deal of medication. In most cases he knows what the medica-tion is for, but in one case he does not. Bruce deals with the complication in fol-lowing the medication routine by ceding authority to his doctor: 'I just do what the man says'. To question the 'man', which for Bruce refers to clinicians who have prescribed the medications, could lead to a difficult process of weighing up evidence. Bruce takes on the classic sick role position as discussed in Chapter 1. Bruce states 'if the doctor says, "that's what you've got to have", fine, have it'. Clinicians are positioned as experts, and trust is placed in those institutions, like medicine and science, that have achieved a status of credible authority in our society. Even if things go wrong under their prescription – as it had with Bruce who had suffered adverse reactions to pharmaceuticals – that trust is not undermined.

Louisa defends her use of medications:

> I come under pressure from other people saying, 'You've been on antide-pressants since 1997, do you think it's a good idea?' And my answer would be, 'Yes' because it has made the difference between functioning and not.

She also has a weekly injection for her multiple sclerosis, and notes that for some people there are difficulties in complying with a regime that requites injec-tions, but for her: 'I wouldn't not do it because the impact of having the medica-tion has been so dramatic.'

Some medications were treated like talismans. For instance, Paula has taken fish oil since she had breast cancer 19 years ago: 'Whether it's done me any good I don't know but they tell me that 19 years is a pretty good record for a person with breast cancer.' She thought 'that's probably mind over matter as well but I still take it … I mean, if people believe in it enough maybe that's part of the way of, you know, fixing it'. Paula is not taking fish oil because it was prescribed by a doctor but because she read an article by a naturopath 'that fish oil is very good for people that have breast cancer'. She has no clear evidence of it working, but she has come to trust in the restorative power of fish oil. Even if the oil itself is not therapeutic, for Paula, the belief itself is therapeutic.

Ingrid described her reliance on medications not in terms of addiction or dependence, but of integration. She had been taking a sleeping pill for about 15 years because 'if I didn't sleep properly I couldn't walk properly and I couldn't work properly … So that's why I've stayed with that and that's probably integrated into my body system now as well as the Amitriptyline'. She believed that she would probably take them 'for the rest of my life, I don't see any reason not to take it'.

As an aside, Ingrid's intervention in the research made me think about the approach I was taking. After I had interviewed Ingrid I gave a seminar presentation at the School of Nursing, Midwifery and Health at Victoria University of Wellington. I notified the people I had interviewed that I would be giving this talk in case any were interested in coming along. Ingrid came along, and although I did not see her after the presentation, a nursing colleague sat beside her in the audience. At the end of my presentation, which was on this topic, Ingrid confided to my colleague that it was all very interesting, but why did it need to be so negative. My colleague conveyed this to me, which provided food for thought. I did not think my presentation had been particularly negative, but it did not focus on the positive approaches that many people took to their health, even in situations where life was made difficult through chronic illness. This made me realise that I should not downplay this positive approach that many people took, hence this particular repertoire of restoring order is one that should not be underemphasised.

In the restorative repertoire, pharmaceuticals are either morally neutral, or are an undoubted good if the medications keep one balanced. The current situation is a 'natural' outcome of some external imposition, summed up by Bruce who says 'shit happens'. For some, like Bruce, there is no responsible agent, so no responsibility is required to consider options and outcomes, as that responsibility is handed over to those who know the best way to deal with the problem or those agents that can have a positive impact. Pharmaceuticalised governance is not problematised, but is integrated with self-identity. Others, like Louisa, do consider the concerns about being governed by drugs, but the cost of not being so governed can be too high.

For some, the negative impact of pharmaceuticals can be emphasised. The 'disordering substances' repertoire captures this, where concerns about drugs are more marked. In this repertoire, pharmaceuticals can be a threat to one's physical or mental equilibrium, but still might be required. People need to take responsibility for pharmaceuticals and, in doing so, might need to 'gamble' on them, weighing up costly risks with benefits. Pharmaceuticals are at times a 'necessary evil', requiring consumers to take a stance of vigilant assessment, a point made back in 1984 by Jon Gabe and Susan Lipshitz-Phillips in relation to benzodiazepines (Gabe and Lipshitz-Phillips 1984). The moral dilemma for patients is in determining whether the cure is worse than the illness, and this is what is being vigilantly assessed. Rather than being able to place trust in the pharmaceutical industry or in health professionals, householders have to make active decisions and take responsibility for them.

In one home, two householders provide two very different but related moral evaluations of pharmaceuticals. Kim, who was on multiple medications that related to, amongst other things, mental illness, stated 'Well, I have these spells where I rebel' against medications that made her 'totally drugged up'. Medications are, in this sense, a form of discipline, but they have side effects of lethargy and weight gain. The consequence of rebelling was to 'Go absolutely high and then crash'. To rebel is to be 'irresponsible'. Her partner, Sophie, articulated a different view. This was partially in response to an earlier interaction between the two. Kim had talked about how she managed the complex routine of medications: 'Once upon a time I used to put them in a weekly supply pack.' At this point, Sophie interrupts with 'Tell the truth, darling ... You used to get me to do it and eventually I said you have to take responsibility for your own bloody medications and not be hand-waited on and that was the end of the weekly pack'. Much later in the interview Sophie returns to the issue of 'responsibility' as an orientation to her concept of health or 'wellness'.

Sophie had been on 'antidepressants and all sorts of stuff and I just weaned myself off'. The concept of 'weaning' relates to ideas of dependency, like a child being dependent on a mother's milk and therefore the mother being responsible for the child. Sophie weaned herself off because she wanted to be 'a functioning member of society ... so in order to get well I had to actually ditch the medication'. For Sophie wellness is being free from medication, taking responsibility for ones-self. The position taken here is contingent: 'They're wonderful things, medicines', but responsibility and ownership of actions are required. When Sophie was asked if she encouraged Kim to take her medicines, she said 'Yes I do ... even though I'm anti mine but we're dealing with different things'. Sophie expresses a view here that there is a moral imperative to be responsible, but there are circumstances where that responsibility cannot be achieved, where it is quite appropriate to take on the sick role and hand over responsibility to external agents – such as pharmaceuticals prescribed by health professionals.

Others have noted that medications can offer a means of control but for some conditions, particularly related to mental health issues, there is ambiguity as 'users of medicine may be both in control and under control' (Whyte *et al.* 2002: 50). For Sophie, taking on the sick role in the case of 'psychological psychiatric type issues' is the responsible thing to do:

taking ownership of it is part of getting well. So you have to take ownership of your own medication, so understand what your medication's doing to you how it's affecting you, be responsible for it.

The earlier exchange between Kim and Sophie over the weekly pack supply is revisited. It is not for Sophie to take responsibility, but for Kim: 'she's got to work out what tablets she needs, make up her own mind to take them and take some responsibility for her own wellbeing'. One can variously be well by taking the responsibility to avoid medication, or be well by taking the responsibility to take 'the damn pills' to prevent intolerable situations. Gareth Williams notes a similar response from patients with rheumatoid arthritis, where they relinquished control over their bodies to doctors but positioned this as a way of achieving independence. Patients did not simply abandon responsibility for their body in a passive way, but controlled what was in their power to control (Williams 1993). A complicated picture of responsibility and dependency, and the social shaping of pharmaceutical practice, is articulated in Kim and Sophie's household.

Other householders had similarly complicated and intense relationships to pharmaceuticals. Viv, for instance, said that: 'I've hated them. I've always hated them ... I've never been a pill taker', but when persuaded to go on to benzodiazepine she 'had to fight and fight and fight to come off them'. Viv provided accounts of the most disorienting side effects of medications, describing one drug (lithium) as 'like the drug from hell', it was 'dreadful ... you wouldn't be aware of what you were doing half the time'. The drug itself is the site of disorder and pathology here, causing disorder in one's very sense of being, turning the participant into a different sort of being, unrecognisable or unknown to herself.

Jasmine, a solo mother with three children in the household, suffered from depression, which was difficult to control, and she had been hospitalised on a number of occasions. Her daughter, who had witnessed her mother's illness, had an ambivalent response to medications: 'if it makes people better I guess it's a good thing'. She said this in front of her mother, perhaps indicating a concern about her mother not taking her medications and the consequences that might have. The daughter later reiterates this ambivalence 'she has to take it so she doesn't really have a choice'.

For Jasmine, there were multiple levels of concern about her medications. Partly this related to adverse consequences of the medication: 'I just worry about what it must do to your insides and your body'. Her daughter chimes in with 'look at all the stuff that's going into her ... it's gross when you think about it'. Another layer of moral concern for Jasmine related to her duties and responsibilities as a mother, and the way in which medication could interfere with that:

I don't like taking it when I've got the children because ... I'm very hard to wake up when I'm on it. Like, it knocks me right out.

Her concern is not waking up in the night if her children are unsettled or distressed: 'Sometimes at night I won't take it, if there's something going on with

Johnnie [her child who has a diagnosis of attention deficit hyperactivity disorder –ADHD] or whatever'. On the other hand, if her children are away 'it can knock me right out and I won't have to worry'. Medications can bring disorder to family roles and a mother's responsibilities. But the consequences of not taking some of her medications can be immediate: 'even just missing that one dose I can feel my heart racing'. There is a clash of responsibilities between the restorative aspects of pharmaceuticals and the care requirements of motherhood.

It was common throughout the interviews to find examples of householders weighing up concerns about side effects with the possible therapeutic value of pharmaceuticals. These side effects fitted into the complex ordering and disordering of medications. Jenny, who has been on long-term dialysis, 'so that's 19 years-worth of prescription drugs', has a 'love/hate relationship with the medications' but she knows she has to take them (Hodgetts *et al.* 2011). When Paula went through her medications she noted that several were for treating side effects from other medications, without raising concerns:

> Now this is a fungicide lozenge because when you're on the chemo tablets you get thrush in your mouth so you've got to suck those. Those are a laxative tablet because once again you have problems when you have all this medication.

However, when she discussed her bottle of sleeping tablets she expressed distaste and stated:

> They started me on one a night and I refused to take one a night because I thought I might get addicted. Because when you're on Prednisone you can't sleep … You've just got so much energy and you can't sleep so they started me on those. Well, I've got a thing about getting addicted to them. I only take half of one at night, of which they're going to get me off them shortly once they get me off this Prednisone.

Her husband did not think she should be concerned about becoming addicted at her age (she was 70), but Paula stated 'I don't want to end up like Michael Jackson'. This concern was to an extent mitigated by her view that if she did not take sleeping pills she would be in a worse position: 'The biggest problem was because I wasn't taking it and getting no sleep then all this medication that they give you to survive doesn't do me any good because you're not sleeping so your body's not getting any rest'. Paula had the complicated task of not only weighing up the risks and benefits of particular medications, but in addition considering the impact of any change she might make on the other medications she was taking.

The moral positioning of householders drawing on a disordering substances repertoire is one of making rational choices based on responsibility and a cost-benefit form of analysis. The moral duty is to be vigilant in maintaining a balance. A form of pharmaceuticalised governance might be necessary, but is nevertheless resisted and, where possible, individual autonomy is promoted.

In the disordering substances repertoire people are required, and do, work to ensure some sense of balance. In the disordering self repertoire, in contrast, pharmaceuticals signify a moral failing of the individual, a stigmatised failing of the body, or both. The focus here is on the failure of the self, and not some particular problem with medications that has to be vigilantly assessed. This failure of the self can be stigmatised by others and lead to forms of discrimination. Access to the requirements to maintain some quality of life can be controlled by others, such as health experts, which can be disempowering. Pharmaceuticals are an inconvenience but they have to be lived with, suggesting a stance of regretful dependence embedded in a pharmaceuticalised form of governance. One's sense of agency is compromised, as one is no longer able to retain control over the self without pharmaceuticals.

Carole's narrative illustrates the disordered body repertoire. Carole had diabetes, sleep apnoea, arthritis, depression, endometriosis and allergic rhinitis. She did not talk to others about her health conditions because of the potential for stigma and discrimination. She associated strong moral evaluations with pharmaceuticals. She was on Metformin for her diabetes, which had side effects that she described as 'not very kind', but it also represented a failure to achieve the self-control required to avoid the drug. She said 'I lost a huge amount of energy and motivation to keep battling the wanting to eat' and 'I just got sick of the effort ... they are definitely a sign of a loss of the sort of drive that I had to keep on top of doing x, y and z ... instead here I am a blob sitting on the couch, yeah and [the medications] are symptoms of it'. Thus, pharmaceuticals are powerful signifiers of failure for Carole.

The moral evaluation of self could change depending on the pharmaceutical. Carole's resistance to taking painkillers for chronic pain positioned her as 'quite good':

> All those kind of drugs are not that great for the stomach ... I try not to take it unless I really have to and I am quite good at managing the pain side of it.

Similarly, Bruce provides a positive moral evaluation of himself for his resistance to painkillers, as he did not 'do that shit'. The avoidance of painkillers relates to a discourse of 'manning up'. This is the same Bruce we met earlier, who takes 'shit loads of medications'. These other medications are not given the same negative moral evaluations that painkillers are given. Notions of 'manning up' were echoed by other men. Justin avoided medications, saying 'I tough it out'. Dave was not taking his prescribed blood pressure pills, arguing that 'if you don't have to take anything it's much better, you feel like you're under your own steam, you're not relying on something else to do what you need to'. The connection between masculinity and a refusal to acknowledge or seek treatment for pain has been noted elsewhere, particularly the construction that the ability to endure pain without help is a key element of masculinity (Courtney 2000; O'Brien *et al.* 2005). Rosaleen O'Brien and colleagues note that this involved people making a distinction between 'minor' or trivial pain, and 'real pain', the latter of which required treatment.

Research undertaken by others shows how medication practices can relate to issues of stigma. HIV researchers found that people would forego medications to avoid disclosing their HIV status in public (Johnston Roberts and Mann 2000). Anne Rogers and colleagues collected accounts from people labelled with schizophrenia who were concerned about being 'discovered' taking medication, as this would indicate their condition (Rogers *et al.* 1998). Carole would go on tramping trips, a common pursuit amongst many people in New Zealand that carries its own positive moral evaluations (Green 2009). She would sometimes share tents with others on these trips. When this happened, she would take her medications quickly 'by the fistful' and not in front of others. She did not want to be seen taking pharmaceuticals and categorised as a pill taker. When she had visitors to her home, she hid her medications from view: 'the vitamins I might have but, no, everything else will be out of sight'. Stigma is attached to prescription medications but not to supplements. Supplements and vitamins do not necessarily disclose a problem that might alter one's life chances, but prescribed medications could.

Information control was essential to avoiding stigmatisation (Gerhardt 1989). Carole does not disclose her many ailments:

> I've seen quite a lot of unintentional bias towards people with medical conditions or disabilities ... I'm dealing with ageism and sexism and that if you add this in, you know, they do impact ... I just keep absolutely quiet about it.

The particular action of medications can provide more or less control for the user, and so could promote or help avoid stigmatisation. The medication for Jasmine's son, who has ADHD, had changed from a pill that had to be taken three times per day to a slow release version he only had to take once in the morning before school. Jasmine said 'so he doesn't have that sort of stigma of going to get the tablet and all the kids knowing'.

The disordered body repertoire positioned the person as dependent on those who provided access to medications. Carole could be frustrated trying to access medications. She provided an anecdote of wanting to build up supplies of Benadryl 'for swine flu because I've got a bit of a higher chance than some of having a few complications' but resented the questions asked at the pharmacy: 'I just object to the third degree'.

The disordered body repertoire connected illness and medication to self-identity. For Louisa, discourses around illness were important, they portrayed the kind of person she was. Her neurologist gets annoyed with her when she contests his view of her as being 'ill'. She states: 'I have an illness but I am not ill', and in fact she could be well, as 'wellness for me isn't the absence of illness, wellness is the ability to lead a full life' even in the face of limitations imposed by illness. She is not able to access laser treatment for her eye because the specialist said he 'can't do anything for her' because of her multiple sclerosis. She thinks she has been classified as a certain 'type' who is ill, and therefore some health professionals do not consider the ways in which particular treatments could add to her quality of life. Louisa does not have a negative moral evaluation of herself as failing, but feels that she is being failed by the moral evaluations of others. The stigmatised self can be a result of internalised or 'felt' stigma, based on a sense of a moral failure of will to sustain a 'natural state', leading to a fall from grace that needs to be hidden from others. Alternatively, it can be a result of 'enacted' stigma, based on the way others, including health professionals, position and respond to you. This stigmatisation of the self may prevent the disclosure of conditions, even to romantic partners, as was the case with 61 per cent of people with epilepsy, found in early research by Scambler and Hopkins (1986).

In this repertoire the focus is on bodily pathology, where medications are a necessary inconvenience and a sign of bodily disorder, signifying a loss of personal control over one's very own body. Medications are themselves neutral, but are a sign of the lowered moral value of the possessor of that body, either in one's own eyes, or a view that others make that judgement of you. Pharmaceuticalised governance unavoidably manifests in everyday life, and this can promote a struggle over the control of one's body and, potentially, conflict with those who are tasked with controlling access to medications. Furthermore, since there was a regretful reliance on pharmaceuticals to obtain a quality of life, hindrances to accessing needed pharmaceuticals were resented. Other obstacles to access noted by householders included the rationing processes of state subsidised pharmaceuticals that made some brands unavailable (to be discussed in Chapter 12). The inability to access some medications because health professionals decided that you would not have an improved quality of life if you took them was another obstacle.

It was from interviewing Carole that the implications of this repertoire powerfully affected me. She was very open about the way medications impacted upon her relationships with others, on the workplace and on her sense of self. The following occurred near the very end of the final interview:

KEVIN: So, has being involved in this made you think differently about anything?
CAROLE: it's made me aware that if I want to stay on top of these things getting into too much detail and thinking too much about all of it is going to have a negative effect.

This, in my research, was a very rare example where the research process appeared to have a negative impact upon the participant in that the act of talking about it added to the burden of illness.

In contrast to the other three repertoires, the disordering society repertoire holds an almost entirely negative view of pharmaceuticals. In this repertoire, pharmaceuticals evoke a society in an unnatural state. People are made anxious by the fear-mongering and marketing of the pharmaceutical industry and the health experts who promote their products. Active resistance to pharmaceutical consumption, or at least passive distancing from consumption, is the stance taken. There is a strong sense of agency in this repertoire where resistance is attainable if one can avoid the disordering effects of a society distanced from nature.

Keith used the photo-elicitation exercise to provide a detailed account that illustrates the disordering society repertoire. A photograph of a radio allowed for reflections on a programme he had heard about Japan's response to swine 'flu', including an 'over the top' reaction of people fleeing a train carriage after someone sneezed. A so-called swine 'flu' epidemic had started in Mexico in 2009 and spread to various parts of the world, appearing intermittently since. Keith interpreted the reported response of Japanese people to the swine 'flu' as:

> Japan being such an industrialised society anyway that what we see here is just another facet of industrialisation through the whole sort of medical, pharmaceutical complex that in fact people are very much embedded within that and that their cultural response was something that could not be separated from that.

He went on to say that Japan 'is very far removed from its natural state' in a 'hyper' industrial complex, and that the 'industrialisation of medicine was something that was very much ingrained culturally within people'. The radio report about Japan is used here by Keith as an illustration of something that he viewed as deeply wrong with society generally, not just restricted to Japanese society. He went on to discuss the contents of the book *In Praise of Slow*, which he had photographed, stating that the book was:

> in praise of low technology. You know, stopping to smell the flowers kind of thing ... the point of the book is to try and make some sort of connection between a sort of an undercurrent of stuff that is deliberately seeking an alternative path forward.

He had taken another photograph of a shelf in his dining room. He noted a contrast between Anti-Flamme (a herbal cream used for bruises and musculoskeletal aches and pains) and an inhaler used by his children for delivering asthma medications. Keith noted that:

> The Anti-Flamme cream – is good stuff. You know, I've had a bad back for the last few weeks and I've been seeing a physio and the Anti-Flamme cream goes a long way, you know, so it's good stuff ... [it] has its place and is something that we regard fondly.

Perhaps because the Anti-Flamme was 'herbal' it was not categorised in a negative way. But when asked what he felt about the inhalers in the photograph, he replied 'I sort of see them as a bit of a prop and a crutch, I suppose, because without them things can go seriously awry'. The inhaler had a 'serious overtone' and is a 'mechanised thing ... plasticated ... belonging to some sort of industry complex'. Later he noted other items in the photograph – photos, birthday cards, a tooth fairy bowl – and said that 'he felt uneasy' about the photograph, with 'that stuff intruding' on personal things. In Keith's evaluation, prescription medicines are positioned as industrial technologies within the context of a society that is disordered and pathological. The medicines signify that something is not right with society, but medicines may be a necessity as a result of society's malaise.

Many householders drew on similar ideas of being distanced from nature. Louisa argued that 'we live in a society where our foods aren't as nutritious as they used to be ... What we eat doesn't match our lifestyle in terms of we eat a high fat, high protein diet and yet we're quite indolent ... We've normalised things that are actually wrong'. As a result of this distancing from nature we increasingly rely on pharmaceuticals. Brett, her partner, chips in with 'You see the ads that come on TV ... we seem to be getting paranoid and the paranoia is probably driven by capitalism's desire to sell, sell, sell', emphasising another pathological influence on pharmaceutical consumption: marketing. Similarly, for Tania pharmaceutical companies played an important disordering role. She suggested that doctors prescribe medications because 'The drug salesman's just been through and said, "Oh, look, we're marketing this and it does this, this and this, here, try some of this"'.

Natasha expressed a concern around a cultural shift where 'you take stuff for everything' and we are 'oversold on how good we can be'. She suggests that unrealistic goals, in terms of being in a permanent state of wellness, are being fostered. Natasha's concern has been well-developed by scholars such as Barbara Marshall (2010), whose critique of a cultural requirement to be forever functional is discussed in Chapter 3. Natasha argued that:

> I live in a world where I don't have to suffer. I don't have to be without. I can buy it for myself. Somebody can help me fix it or whatever [it is] based on, perfect health or perfect bodies or perfect lives, that's all tied up in a commercial world of transaction ... we're constantly being bombarded with advertising and media and marketing and selling, selling, selling.

Natasha then took a slightly different view, saying:

> when you think of any number of things that can go wrong with the human body, then if you tried to cure or fix or cut off everything before it happened, you'd be wrapped up in cotton wool somewhere. So it's the risk aversion stuff, the safety stuff that goes along with that, that whole safety culture.

A culture of risk aversion, and the promotion of anxiety around illness, happiness and functioning perfectly, made Natasha suspicious of medications. Verity offered similar sentiments, stating that: 'I think we've decreased our resistance, we're trying to make life too clean and at the same time we're weakening our own resistance to ... what's naturally out there'.

In many ways we can see these householders drawing on the kinds of concepts developed within sociology, such as medicalisation and its drivers discussed in the previous chapter, and broader critiques related to forms of social organisation in industrialised capitalist societies. In this repertoire, pharmaceuticals signify a distancing from a more natural world. They can be a prop to deal with the unnatural state we are in, but ideally they should be resisted. They can potentially be resisted in situations where the 'self' is not reliant or dependent on medications, or where disease and illness are viewed as natural and not to be avoided, allowing resistance to pharmaceuticalised forms of governance where quality of life is dependent on external medical agents. Illness results from 'upstream' social and cultural influences. Pharmaceuticals only deal with the symptoms, and so as a society we are morally obliged to consider social and cultural change to restore order.

## Conclusion

A goal of this chapter has been to demonstrate how relationships between people and forms of social organisation can be governed in relation to pharmaceuticals. The focus has been on governance at an interpersonal and subjective level, where one's sense of self and one's understandings of the responsibility for both the cause of disease and how to respond to disease and ill health influence our conduct. Our relationship to pharmaceuticals influences our life chances, not just in the sense of whether they have therapeutic value that may extend life, or in the case of adverse reactions to pharmaceuticals leading to premature death or other ailments, they additionally influence our life chances in terms of how we might be categorised and what sort of stigma is associated with different categories.

This typology of repertoires was something that we developed from the analysis and interpretation of the interviews with householders, but of course there are many other researchers who have explored the social meanings and moral positioning that people take in relation to medications. For example, early research by Jon Dowell and Harriet Hudson indicated how medications, along with illness, can challenge our sense of identity (Dowell and Hudson 1997). Nicky Britten suggested that people who attended primary care practices could be categorised in two broad ways: as those who justified their actions on the basis of medical opinion; and those who provided unorthodox accounts that viewed medications as unnatural (Britten 1996). As such, Britten identified that people make quite different moral evaluations of medication practices.

There is no last word here on some definitive picture of the moral forces at play in relation to medication consumption. Different researchers provide their own insights. One particular insight that I came to in this research was that the concept of pharmaceuticalised governance could be useful not only for under-standing processes of acceptance of, and resistance to, medication recommenda-tions, but also how intertwined medication practices are with moral evaluations. The following chapter furthers the exploration of subjective and interpersonal aspects of pharmaceuticalised governance by looking at how medications are used in the home.

## References

Britten, N. (1996). Lay views of drugs and medicine: Orthodox and unorthodox accounts. In: *Modern Medicine: Lay Perspectives and Experiences* (eds S.J. Williams and M. Calnan), 48–73. London: UCL Press.

Courtney, W. (2000). Constructions of masculinity and their influence on men's well-being: A theory of gender and health. *Social Science and Medicine* 50 (10): 1385–1401.

Dew, K., Norris, P., Gabe, J., Chamberlain, K. and Hodgetts, D. (2015). Moral discourses and pharmaceuticalised governance in households. *Social Science and Medicine* 131: 272–279.

Dowell, J. and Hudson, H. (1997). A qualitative study of medication-taking behaviour in primary care. *Family Practice* 14 (5): 369–375.

Gabe, J. and Lipshitz-Phillips, S. (1984). Tranquillisers as social control? *The Socio-logical Review* 32 (3): 524–546.

Gerhardt, U. (1989). *Ideas about Illness: An Intellectual and Political History of Medical Sociology*. Basingstoke: Macmillan.

Gilbert, N. and Mulkay, M. (1984). *Opening Pandora's Box: A Sociological Analysis of Scientists' Discourse*. Cambridge: Cambridge University Press.

Green, J. (2009). 'Walk this way': Public health and the social organization of walking. *Social Theory and Health* 7 (1): 20–38.

Hodgetts, D., Chamberlain, K., Gabe, J., Dew, K., Radley, A., Madden, H., Norris, P. and Nikora, L. (2011). Emplacement and everyday use of medications in domestic dwell-ings. *Health and Place* 17 (1): 353–360.

Johnston Roberts, K. and Mann, T. (2000). Barriers to antiretroviral medication adher-ence in HIV-infected women. *AIDS Care* 12 (4): 377–386.

Lemke, T. (2001). 'The birth of bio-politics': Michel Foucault's lecture at the Collége de France on neo-liberal governmentality. *Economy and Society* 30 (2): 190–207.

Marshall, B.L. (2010). Science, medicine and virility surveillance: 'Sexy seniors' in the pharmaceutical imagination. *Sociology of Health and Illness* 32 (2): 211–224.

O'Brien, R., Hunt, K. and Hart, G. (2005). 'It's caveman stuff, but that is to a certain extent how guys still operate': Men's accounts of masculinity and help seeking. *Social Science and Medicine* 61: 503–516.

Rogers, A., Day, J.C., Williams, B., Randall, F., Wood, P., Healy, D. and Bentall, R.P. (1998). The meaning and management of neuroleptic medication: A study of patients with a diagnosis of schizophrenia. *Social Science and Medicine* 47 (9): 1313–1323.

Scambler, G. and Hopkins, A. (1986). Being epileptic: Coming to terms with stigma. *Sociology of Health and Illness* 8 (1): 26–43.

Taylor, S. and Ashworth, C. (1987). Durkheim and social realism: An approach to health and illness. In: *Sociological Theory and Medical Sociology* (ed. G. Scambler), 37–58. London: Tavistock.

Whyte, S.R., Van der Geest, S. and Hardon, A. (2002). *Social Lives of Medicines.* New York: Cambridge University Press.

Williams, G. (1993). Chronic illness and the pursuit of virtue in everyday life. In: *Worlds of Illness: Biographical and Cultural Perspectives on Health and Disease* (ed. A. Radley), 92–108. London and New York: Routledge.

# 5 Medication practices in the home

## Introduction

A wealth of medications is likely to be found in any household. They may get into the house by various means. They may be prescribed by a general practitioner (GP), recommended by an alternative health practitioner or some other health professional. They may be purchased from supermarkets, pharmacies or ordered online. They may be given to householders by relatives, friends or work colleagues. Once inside the house they can be kept in many different places: the bathroom, bedside cabinets, the pantry, on shelves or counters in kitchens and lounges. They may be in coat pockets, handbags or in the glove box of the car in the garage. Medications are everywhere and we encounter them regularly.

As noted in the previous chapter, when we conducted our research on householders' use of medications we asked our householder participants to draw maps of their home and point out where they kept their medications. Then we asked them, if they were happy with the idea, to bring their medications out so we could talk about them. For many households this was quite an onerous task. Medications were hauled out from all directions, and placed before us on the kitchen table or the lounge floor. The medication-elicitation interviews provided us with a wealth of information and a delightful array of stories that we could ponder and relate to our academic interests.

Some things were immediately striking in this process. One was the sheer amount of medication that people found in their homes and the surprise that many expressed when they saw them all in one spot. When Tania was asked if she would bring all her medications out she said 'Oh, God. Right, well, put your feet up' noting that she had this 'huge pile'. For some participants they were disconcerted that they had so much medication and expressed a desire to get rid of some of it. When all the medications in the house were put on her kitchen table Bev turned to her husband saying 'we have to sort this out, it's embarrassing' (Hodgetts *et al.* 2011). For others there was a surprise that they had so many medications that were out of date. Natasha expressed a sense of guilt when finding out that she had expired medications: 'oopsy'. But for all of them, they were able to tell us stories that gave us a sense of the kinds of relationships that people developed and sustained around medications. People use medications in ways that connects them to others and link them 'to health professionals beyond the walls of the house and networks of relationships surrounding the procurement, storage, and construction of medications in the therapeutic spaces of the home' (Hodgetts *et al.* 2011).

These connections influence how we think about medications, what we do with them, and how much of our medication practices we reveal to others.

In making therapeutic choices people have to make decisions about who they trust, and what they trust (Fainzang 2017). This issue of trust relates to what we can call legitimacy: what medication practices do we consider to be legitimate? When we answer this question, we are revealing what and who we trust. There has been a great deal of interest in the relationship between trust and expertise in sociology. Anthony Giddens defines trust as:

> a device for stabilizing interaction. To be able to trust another person is to be able to rely upon that person to produce a range of anticipated responses.
>
> (Giddens 1987: 136)

We are forced to trust when we have a lack of information. This occurs in many situations in our everyday lives, and is a common experience in relation to health issues. We know little about the medicines we consume, whether 'natural' or synthetic. I put natural in quote marks to trouble the category, as most natural products – herbs, supplements and so on – are assembled in ways that we know little about. We are heavily reliant on experts and on complex processes. We depend upon specialists to provide advice on how best to manage ourselves in relation to these systems (Giddens 1991). Giddens (1991) argues that 'manufactured uncertainty' and 'manufactured risk' are central elements of contemporary society. These elements have their origin in the prevalence of science, technology and industry which, in effect, 'disembed' social relations from the contexts of action. What that means is that our relationships of trust are extended way beyond those with whom we have actual contact. Important relationships are less likely to be established through face-to-face encounters, but are increasingly with people at a distance, or who are anonymous. In the case of pharmaceuticals these people at a distance may include scientists in research institutions, CEOs of drug companies, members of drug regulatory committees, and those handling the storage and distribution of drugs. Due to the complexity of the many systems that we have created to aid and assist our lives, individuals cannot possibly understand or control all the forces that affect them. In other words, we have to invest a great deal of trust in vicarious relationships, with a vast range of people, when we do something as simple as put a pill in our mouths.

Patrick Brown and Michael Calnan (2010) suggest that, as the pharmaceutical industry is largely faceless, trust issues are significant. One strategy to combat a lack of trust in the industry is the use of substantial resources by drug companies to influence patients and health care professionals, as discussed in Chapters 3 and 8. Drug companies gaining the trust of health professionals is especially important, as Brown and Calnan suggest that the drug prescribing health professionals play an important role as mediators between drug companies and patients. Medical professionals are likely to be trusted by patients whereas patients might not so easily bestow trust on anonymous drug company personnel. The medical professionals themselves, by necessity, place trust in a range of other institutional players, such as those agencies that regulate pharmaceutical products, journals that publish research results on drug trials, those who are tasked with educating health professionals and so on (Brown and Calnan 2010). As noted throughout this book, these sources may not always be trustworthy either.

Trust is a necessary result of our inability to be fully informed about science and technology. We have to place trust in experts in these areas. But many people are sceptical about the claims to specialist knowledge of scientific experts. Because of this ambivalence, trust in experts is fragile. Giddens suggests that, in fact, there is a constant tension between experts and officials on the one hand, and lay actors on the other, over the appropriation of knowledge (Giddens 1991). That is, there is tension between people who are designated as health experts and people who seek health support over what forms of knowledge and what sorts of actions in relation to health are allowable and given credibility. By looking at the way people use medications in the household, we can see these issues of trust and credibility play out in ways that are usually hidden from view.

In working through the data that we collected in households, I was struck by the kinds of activities that householders undertook in overseeing the use of medications. There were many decisions to make, and householders undertook careful observation of themselves or of their family members to gauge the effects of medication. Were the medications working? Did they cause unanticipated problems? Many of our participants experimented with their medications, considering the right dose for them, or the right combination. Homes, therefore, were not so different from the science laboratory, but with ideas about what kinds of experiment to perform coming in from all sorts of sources. Somehow our participants had to weigh all this up and decide upon a therapeutic strategy.

When I was immersed in all this analysis, as mentioned in Chapter 1, I started reading a book by Anders Blok and Torben Jensen (2011) titled: *Bruno Latour: Hybrid Thoughts in a Hybrid World*. I had long enjoyed Latour's work, liking his provocations as they got me to think hard about many things, but I had not thought about using Latour in this research. However, reading Blok and Jensen reminded me of Latour's use of the concept of hybrid, and I began to think that this could be quite a useful concept when applied to our material. I shared this idea with my research colleagues and they were very enthusiastic – so I got to writing. When I shared the writing with others and received their input, one of my colleagues suggested that I could use Michel de Certeau's ideas, particularly his use of the concepts of tactics. I had only had a passing acquaintance with his work but always thought it was something I should know more about – so off I went to the library. These two approaches, of Latour and de Certeau, combined really well and helped me to consider the home as an active therapeutic centre, but one that often hybridised the content and form of other centres. To consider the home as a therapeutic centre shifts our understanding of the role of health professionals and of the agency of patients. This interpretation suggests that the clinics of health professionals are not the centres of therapeutic practice, but are one source, albeit an important source, of advice and therapy for the clinic/home hybrid (Dew 2016; Dew *et al.* 2014).

Thinking of the home as a therapeutic centre signals ways in which the household cuts across primary and secondary care, mainstream and alternative practices. The home links a wide array of networks, including family, friends, libraries, the Internet and the whole range of health advisors. The breadth and depth of connections and activities are assimilated in the home, and the form of this assimilation is influenced by internal household relationships.

Before exploring medication practices in the home, I will outline some of the concepts used by Latour and de Certeau that we found particularly fruitful. Latour makes the argument that what he calls 'the moderns' are a type of people who maintain a belief in the existence of pure categories, seen in the headings of daily newspapers: 'Economy, Politics, Science, Books, Culture, Religion and Local Events', but at the same time 'all of culture and all of nature get churned up again every day' (Latour 1993: 2) in the form of 'unruly hybrids' (Blok and Jensen 2011: 55). That is, in everyday life and in social practice these categories are not neatly separated out. Households can be seen as hybrids mixing up and reassembling the pure categories from other health practice spaces, such as the office of the mainstream medical practitioner or the consulting rooms of the alternative healer. In the offices and consulting rooms of health professionals efforts are made to separate out various domains, such as science from non-science, orthodox from unorthodox and natural from artificial or synthetic. However, these get mixed up in household spaces where responses to illness and well-being involve pragmatic decision-making based on what seems to work or what might work, rather than purified rule-following.

Households engage in their own form of truth production through research, experimentation and observation. The use of the term 'truth' here is somewhat challenging, as from this sort of perspective it is difficult, if not impossible, to determine a single truth. Truth is relative. It varies from site to site and from situation to situation. From this Latourian perspective, something like 'truth' and something like 'belief' cannot be easily delineated. I will continue to use the term 'truth production', but if you are uncomfortable with that you could perhaps substitute the term 'belief production'. I don't want to force my epistemological assumptions on to you.

Gareth Williams and Jennie Popay contend that lay beliefs pose little direct challenge to the power of the medical profession because they 'remain outside the worlds of science and politics' (Williams and Popay 1994: 118) and are disorganised. This is an understandable view, but we can look at this another way: lay beliefs and practices are inherently a challenge to the power of medicine, particularly because they are not readily visible and therefore not readily disciplined. They are not overseen by those with expertise and those with authority. They are not controlled by some governing group, such as a medical council, or a government agency that oversees the safe use of medications. Latour refers to these kinds of governing groups as centres of calculation. These centres of calculation are undermined in the home, where the products of calculation, such as the medical prescription, the clinical advice and the regimens of well-being are reworked and re-formed. Medical practices are positioned by governing groups as scientific practices, and therefore have to be uncontaminated by other practices that are not regarded as scientific. Medicine has to be, in Latour's term, purified. The work of purification of scientific medical practice is hybridised in the daily activities of householders enacting wellness.

For Latour, a centre of calculation is able to coordinate scientific practices that are widely spread, both in terms of time and space (Latour 2005). We could consider a medical council as a centre of calculation in this sense. The council members meet at one site, but their decisions and oversight of health professionals' standards are widely spread, shaping practices in many consultation rooms and clinics. The centre of calculation can bind many sites to it through such activities as evidence-based practice, quality assurance and practice guidelines (as discussed in Chapter 2) enacted through the various medical councils, colleges and schools. There are guidelines on different conditions and what to prescribe, at what dose and what sort of oversight is required. If practitioners do not follow the prescribed guidelines they may be disciplined, audited and monitored. That is, there is a great deal of effort that goes in to standardising the actions of health professionals so that they conform to ideals of practice. By standardising practices, the centre of calculation gains control over the actions of others, even where those others are at a distance (Latour 1988, 1992). For the medical elites, power is gained by developing treatment guidelines that all practitioners can follow and which can be applied to whole categories of patients. The medical profession can thus, control many practices from one place – but households decentre and unravel these binds. Homes are sites where wellness and remedy is performed and not directly overseen by centres of calculation (there are some exceptions to this, including home visits to administer medications to confused elderly patients).

De Certeau's work provides other insights. De Certeau's concern is with analysing the 'micro-subversive tactics in the practice of everyday life' (Ward 2000: 8). His approach encourages us to attend to the practices of people in relation to established rules and ideas (de Certeau 1984). People are not passive in relation to dominant ways of thinking or acting (sometimes described as norms or dominant discourses) or externally imposed rules of operation, but actively and tactically engage with them. In this chapter, we look at some of the active processes of production of medication practices in a space that is generally hidden from view and where medications are assumed to be passively consumed. Householders make 'innumerable and infinitesimal transformations of and within the dominant cultural economy in order to adapt it to their own interests and their own rules' (de Certeau 1984: xiv).

The concepts of hybrids and tactics illuminate the networked nature of household medication practices, and how these re-assemble and subvert externally imposed norms and dominant discourses. By relating the concepts of hybrids and tactics to that of trust, we can consider the ways that health and well-being practices achieve credibility. This analysis has implications for health practitioners, as what is said and done in the clinic is translated in unanticipated ways when patients go home. Decision-making is not a one-off occurrence made in the disciplined and monitored spaces of the clinic.

In the rest of this chapter, the activities of diagnosis and prescribing in the home will be addressed. In the following chapter, the sources of the practices undertaken in the household will be explored.

### *Diagnosing and prescribing*

Diagnosing and prescribing were common activities in households, and not something reserved solely for health professionals. Householders may not have the practice, expertise and particular skills of clinicians (Prior 2003) and their understandings may conflict with those of medical science (Fainzang 2017), but they are regular diagnosticians. In developing a treatment plan, householders observe, experiment, assess, draw on a range of advice and self-prescribe. Householders deviate from or reject advice and develop their own expertise. A critical dimension of diagnostic activity is to determine when outside help is required. Annemarie Jutel notes that before any encounter with a health professional, a patient makes a premedical assessment (Jutel 2011). Close observation and the identification of the 'normal' are central elements in determining the severity of conditions. This can be for minor conditions, seen in one of our participants, Natasha, when describing her decision not to take her daughter to a doctor, as 'she's not [got], you know, green mucous or anything so probably no infection'. It can be for more severe conditions, seen in Hazel's decision not to take her fevered child to the GP, where there have been past concerns about febrile seizures, 'because I know that that's the way she gets sick'. Hazel is combining her own medical understandings and past experience with observations to make a diagnosis, to consider a prognosis and a treatment plan. Febrile seizures are a worrying possibility, but from her careful observation over time Hazel distinguishes between types of fever. Householders can be acutely sensitive to the nature of the conditions of others who share their homes, identifying what is normal and abnormal for themselves and for those around them, and then determining a course of action based on that identification.

Professional expertise was not usually a first resort, and self-prescribing was a feature of home wellness practices. As Fleur's son Jason stated: 'we don't go seeking help straight away'. He ridicules professional advice: 'when I know I've got a sore throat I don't want to go and pay somebody to tell me I've got a sore throat'. Payment of primary care services varies from country to country, and in New Zealand, where this data was collected, patients have to pay to see their GP. Trystan, Jason's brother, had been given a diagnosis of gout by his doctor, but according to Trystan the doctor just wanted to keep doing blood tests so Trystan decided to self-prescribe, which entailed modifying his diet. Many households use what could be termed folk remedies. When asked if there were any household remedies used for 'sore throats and things' Jessica's household collectively listed lemon, honey and ginger tea, salt and water, and baking soda for 'upset stomachs and things like that'. Recommended prescriptions from outside the household could be supplemented with other therapeutic interventions, such as antibiotics with self-prescribed probiotics or high doses of vitamin C.

Householders commonly deviated from the recommendations of others, whether orthodox or unorthodox, tactically engaging with these recommendations and adapting them to their own interests and rules (de Certeau 1984). Deviations included stopping medications, rejecting medications and ignoring warnings. In one interview, Sylvia noted in a critical tone that there was an unfinished packet of antibiotics amongst her household's medications. Her husband, Dan, defended this egregious action of not completing his course of antibiotics by saying 'it was probably a case of if I forgot to take it for a day and then there was no point in trying to just restart the course'. Dan draws on his own understanding of how antibiotics work as a defence for his actions. Ideally one should follow the rules prescribed by the centres of calculation and take the whole course of antibiotics, but if this gets disrupted he has to make a decision about what the best course of action is, and so he alters the prescribed treatment plan. Dan makes this decision on his own without consulting a health professional.

Dave talks about his family's partiality for a non-prescribed cold medication – Lemsip. He says:

> whenever we have it we have it with a bit of rum and honey as well. Because it says on the side of the box, 'Danger: you're not supposed to have with alcohol'. That's the bit of spice in our life.

When asked to justify his disregard of the prohibition against alcohol, Dave says the alcohol 'enhances the whole experience really', and he is not concerned about any negative effects 'because I don't think it's very dangerous, I think it's just kind of a lemon drink'. Dave also resists his doctor's advice to take blood pressure pills, kept in the bathroom, because he does not think he needs them, 'so as a result of that I kind of forget' to take them. Dave tactically forgets rather than outright refuses, but the result is the same as the blood pressure pills remain in the bathroom cupboard.

Prescribed medications could be stopped because of fear of side effects or a view that there were better alternatives. Tania was concerned about the adverse effects of the GP-prescribed blood-thinning medication Warfarin for 'clots on my lungs' so she 'stopped taking it'. Tania also stopped taking a prescribed diuretic as 'it's better to just drink water and that flushes it through and have parsley tea and stuff – natural diuretics'. Tania is actively engaged in devising her own treatment plan, taking advice from outside the home but altering and hybridising that advice. Because she was getting bad stomach pains from taking medication to prevent osteoporosis, Paula has 'sort of put that on hold in the meantime'; a decision she made by herself without discussion with her GP. Bethany was taking a painkiller for her back injury 'but I just felt it put me on a trip and I absolutely hated it'.

Decisions about whether or not to take a drug could be based on the impacts of its effects on one's everyday activities. Paula and her husband have a pill container they put out at breakfast time. She did not take a prescribed diuretic from this container one day because she was going out, and the pill 'being a diuretic you have to keep running to the loo all the time'. She had not disclosed to her GP that this was how she managed the situation, suggesting that 'I don't think … the odd day hurts not to take it because the next day I will take it'. She has come to this conclusion on her own, without any discussion with other health professionals.

Ingrid takes a prescribed sleeping pill, but she does not tell her Ayurveda practitioner:

> because he'd likely have a heart attack. He can't believe that somebody would have a problem with not sleeping.

In this instance Ingrid is deviating from the recommendations of an alternative practitioner to follow more conventional advice. By contrast, Janice provides an account of having bowel problems and her doctor suggesting 'basically don't eat anything that's going to stimulate your bowel and then just do it manually every day by using an enema'. Janice did not pursue this advice, instead following the advice of her naturopath to take an appetite stimulant, which she keeps in the pantry. Ingrid and Janice are determining who to trust in relation to the specific problem they are addressing. This does not mean they distrust the other practitioner whose advice that they are not following in this instance; they obviously go to both practitioners. Their decisions are more refined: they are deciding who to trust in the particular situation they are in, for the particular problem they are confronting.

Householders hybridise wellness practices, taking some suggestions from different places and recombining them in relation to their own understandings. Fainzang provides an example of how householders can mix up therapeutic approaches in her own research. Josiane is prescribed a drug by her medical doctor but has the drug tested by an alternative practitioner to decide if the drug is the right one for her (Fainzang 2017). Janice makes decisions in the home to reject medications, even after collecting the suggested medication from the pharmacist. Tania says that a medication to prevent acid reflux 'stops the … production of acid but then if you don't have acid it doesn't digest your food'. She makes a decision to reduce the prescribed dose as 'I get a problem with processing protein'.

Decisions about expiry dates are made in the home. Such decisions could be based on the value placed on the medication by the householder, rather than the 'expert' advice on the bottle. For Jessica, an asthma drug used for her children kept in the household first aid kit 'that you can't actually get any more' is out of date, but 'it's like precious cargo' and 'will still be alright'. Dave contests the claims about expiry on a cough mixture: 'I can't believe anything would ever be a problem with that'. Zoe, who positions herself as a hoarder, has older medications packed neatly in a box: 'I find it hard to chuck stuff out'. She will use antibiotics that have gone past the use by date for her bad cough. Erica looks at one medication for pain relief, saying:

> It's from December 2008. Oh well, it still works! [laughs] If I drop over dead somebody's just going to have to go through my medicine cabinet and say, 'Oh, no wonder, Diclofenac's passed its due date'.

Householders used a number of strategies to justify ignoring the expiry date claims on their medications – including irony, disbelief and a cost-benefit or risk-benefit assessment. Some other householders stuck to the letter of the law, using the interview process to identify expired medications and throwing them out.

Some householders become experts. Some householders are systematic, basing household therapeutics on particular approaches, such as the use of homeopathy or aromatherapy. Householders could gain expertise in these areas by taking courses, joining organisations and undertaking a concerted course of reading. The development of expertise in the household so that trust did not have to be placed in others was much more common in the past, and is less likely to be encountered today. For example, in the later 1800s and early 1900s, homeopathic practitioners and pharmacists prepared domestic kits for their patients with directions for the administration of remedies so that patients could treat themselves. Patients would therefore have to diagnose and determine what prescription was right. By 1890, over 1 million of these had been sold in the United States (Kaufman 1988). Homeopaths and herbalists could go even further than this by encouraging patients to prepare their own remedies (Belgrave 1985). In only a few households do we see the exercise of this level of expertise and control.

Householders may take on expertise in relation to orthodox biomedicine, sometimes out of necessity. For Hazel, developing expertise was necessary, because she was not able to fully trust health professionals to look out for her even though she has been recorded as being 'allergic to some antibiotics' and 'could die' if she took them again. She told the prescribing doctor:

> I'm allergic to sulphur and he looked at my notes and said, 'It's not in here that you're allergic to sulphur', which made me a little bit upset because I've been going to that practice for a long time ... but that's why I'm always insistent myself. I take it upon myself because I don't ... it's not that I don't trust doctors – sometimes I don't – but I just think I've got to take responsibility for that one, since it is so serious.

This example illustrates a requirement for intense self-surveillance in some situations, and the importance of prescribing expertise by householders. Trust is provisionally made: it can be withdrawn or restored, it is not static.

Householders can become experts through their own training and through necessity, but also through processes of experimentation to determine such things as the right dose for them, when to take medications and when not to. Ingrid knew that if she took too much vitamin C 'it gives you diarrhoea, that's how you know so you don't do that'. Louisa's experimentation was due to her view that 'I take an awful lot of medications and I want to be sure that the medications I'm taking are the medications that I need to take'. She was taking a homeopathic medication for urinary tract infection (UTI):

> I got to three drops once a day then I started having UTIs so I did four drops once a day. Hallelujah, it seemed to work so I left it at that.

Louisa did something similar to determine the right level of prescribed medication. Because 'anti-depressants get a bad rap' she tried to get her dose down, 'and by the time I'd got down to having 20 mg a day I was an absolute mess' – so in consultation with her doctor she increased her dose again.

Self-observation commonly led to the rejection of particular medications. Zoe took a herbal preparation she described as a 'sugar killer' for weight loss, stating that: 'It puts you off everything. Didn't work'. Mark rejected a remedy for his joint problems because 'I tried that but I didn't notice any difference so I didn't buy anymore'. Louisa had a prescription from a homeopath 'but I didn't find it helpful'. A process of trial, error and retrial is common in households. Dan had tried 'just about everything' for his hay fever, and a pharmacist recommendation was not only the cheapest but the most effective. Hazel stated that she 'experimented a lot' noting that she took supplements at times, homeopathic medicines and 'even more extreme things and herbs and Chinese herbs'.

In our 55 households there were numerous other stories of experimentation. Householders choose what medicines to use, to find the right dose and to find the best time to take them. Householders engaged in a considerable amount of such experimentation to determine what they considered to be best practice for themselves.

Some householders are well aware of the difficulties of determining causes from simple observation. Avril did not want to take antibiotic cream for rosacea so she tried 'a strange mixture of herbs'. Her condition improved, but she stated:

> I don't know if it's the change of season but my rosacea (a skin condition with a red facial rash) is much less bad than it was. It was all lumpy and now it's gone smooth. So whether or not it was related to that Chinese herb I don't know.

Similarly, she stated that after taking a homeopathic remedy for hay fever, where she was 'sneezing really terribly', she subsequently:

[D]idn't have any trouble for the rest of the day. Whether or not it was that or it was just coincidence but anyway, it seemed worth it for the sugar pill or whatever it is [laughter].

Coincidence, and the idea of a sugar pill, is given some weight as possible explanations here. The sugar pill phrase is referring to the idea of the placebo effect, a well-known and common argument used to explain why people get benefit from unproven remedies (see Chapter 1 for discussion of the placebo). This ambivalence is further played out as Avril refers to another homeopathic remedy where she 'didn't notice any difference whatsoever'. So Avril self-observes and notes changes, whilst remaining cautious about attributing positive effects to the alternative medications she tries, although she is more emphatic in noting when they do not work. I suggest that Avril is providing a defence against common discourses about alternative therapies, that they are quackery and only gullible people use them. Avril is indicating that alternative medicine has an effect on her, but she is not going to be categorised as someone who is easily persuaded. She is not gullible.

In the examples provided so far, views on wellness practices tend to align within households, but this is not always the case. Janice notes different approaches to medication in her household: her son prefers a Nurofen for a headache, but Janice would prefer him to have 'a drink of water first, because I think hydration is a huge thing with headaches'. In relation to her son's prescribed medications, she says 'he's still quite blindly, "Well, it's a doctor, they know" whereas Sam's had a few ups and downs and he's more, "I'll tough it out"'. Janice, the mother, takes opportunities to ask questions, gauge developments and offer advice, whilst at the same time responding to the different orientations her children have towards medications and health professionals.

Janice's considered responses to her children's perspectives manifest the care and love that can surround medication practices. Care can take many forms, including care to ensure that routines are established when the demands of pharmaceutical consumption become complicated. Spaces in homes are used strategically. Medications are placed carefully so that they act as reminders, and to establish routines around consumption (Hodgetts *et al.* 2011). Care may involve badgering or reminding partners, children or parents to take their medications. Ensuring loved ones follow their medication routines may involve adult children moving closer to elderly parents, or bringing their parents into their home so that their medication practices can be overseen (Hodgetts *et al.* 2011).

## Concluding comments

Pharmaceuticalisation is ubiquitous. Every household in our research had a mixture of prescribed and self-selected pharmaceuticals and medications, even households that placed a strong emphasis on alternative therapeutic approaches. The medical profession had a strong presence in households, but its influence was not always a dominant factor in pharmaceuticalised social practices, and pharmaceuticals could be used in ways unanticipated by health professionals.

Pharmaceutical practices in the home, through the observation of others and the establishment of routine, shape relationships between householders and manifest the love and care within homes. Diagnosis and prescription practices in the household have to occur as householders determine who, if anyone, needs to be consulted and when; how to handle untoward effects of prescribed medications; and how to reconcile advice from alternative sources and with their own experiences, observations and understandings. These practices can vary from the advice provided by outside experts, with advice being supplemented, modified or rejected and through this householders can challenge what is expected of them. The health expertise found in consulting rooms, Internet sites and pharmacies is decentred as householders develop their own hierarchies of sources based on combinations of experience, worldview and the particular issue they are trying to resolve and how that issue responds to their attempts at resolution.

Through observation and experimentation, households are sites of truth production; and by varying, rejecting and combining recommendations, we can see householders drawing on norms but manipulating them to their own ends. Using the concept of hybrids in a Latourian sense, and taking as central de Certeau's perspective on the productive capacities of everyday life, householders should not be seen as passive consumers of dominant discourses but as active producers of hybridised medication practices beyond the purview of medicine's centres of calculation. The following chapter further explores the networked and hybrid nature of households' wellness practices by examining the sources for these practices.

## References

Belgrave, M. (1985). 'Medical men' and 'lady doctors': The making of a New Zealand profession, 1867–1941. PhD dissertation. Victoria University of Wellington.

Blok, A. and Jensen, T. (2011). *Bruno Latour: Hybrid Thoughts in a Hybrid World.* London and New York: Routledge.

Brown, P. and Calnan, M. (2010). Braving a faceless new world? Conceptualizing trust in the pharmaceutical industry and its products. *Health* 16 (1): 57–75.

de Certeau, M. (1984). *The Practice of Everyday Life.* Berkeley: University of California Press.

Dew, K. (2016). Purifying and hybridising categories in healthcare decision-making: The clinic, the home and the multidisciplinary team. *Health Sociology Review* 25 (2): 142–156.

Dew, K., Chamberlain, K., Hodgetts, D., Norris, P., Radley, A. and Gabe, J. (2014). Home as a hybrid centre of medication practice. *Sociology of Health and Illness* 36 (1): 28–43.

Fainzang, S. (2017). *Self-Medication and Society: Mirages of Autonomy.* Abingdon: Routledge.

Giddens, A. (1987). *Social Theory and Modern Sociology.* Stanford: Stanford University Press.

Giddens, A. (1991). Structuration theory: Past, present and future. In: *Theory of Structuration: A Critical Appreciation of Giddens* (eds C. Bryant and D. Jary), 201–221. London: Routledge.

Hodgetts, D., Chamberlain, K., Gabe, J., Dew, K., Radley, A., Madden, H., Norris, P. and Nikora, L. (2011). Emplacement and everyday use of medications in domestic dwellings. *Health and Place* 17 (1): 353–360.

Jutel, A. (2011). *Putting a Name to It: Diagnosis in Contemporary Society*. Baltimore: The Johns Hopkins University Press.

Kaufman, M. (1988). Homeopathy in America: The rise and fall and persistence of a medical heresy. In: *Other Healers: Unorthodox Medicine in America* (ed. N. Gevitz), 99–123. Baltimore: Johns Hopkins University Press.

Latour, B. (1988). The politics of explanation: An alternative. In: *Knowledge and Reflexivity: New Frontiers in the Sociology of Knowledge* (ed. S. Woolgar), 154–176. London: Sage.

Latour, B. (1992). The costly ghastly kitchen. In: *The Laboratory Revolution in Medicine* (eds A. Cunningham and W. Perry), 295–303. Cambridge: Cambridge University Press.

Latour, B. (1993). *We Have Never Been Modern*. Cambridge, MA: Harvard University Press.

Latour, B. (2005). *Reassembling the Social: An Introduction to Actor-Network-Theory*. New York: Oxford.

Prior, L. (2003). Belief, knowledge and expertise: The emergence of the lay expert in medical sociology. *Sociology of Health and Illness* 25: 41–57.

Ward, G. (2000). Introduction. In: *The Certeau Reader* (ed. G. Ward), 1–14. Oxford: Blackwell.

Williams, G. and Popay, J. (1994). Lay knowledge and the privilege of experience. In: *Challenging Medicine* (eds J. Gabe, D. Kelleher and G. Williams), 118–139. London: Routledge.

# 6  Sources of practices and their contestation

In the previous chapter, the therapeutic practices that occur in the home were discussed. These practices are developed in relation to sources of information and advice that come from outside the home. Householders have to determine what advice to put their faith in, and in so doing develop hierarchies of advisors. They additionally draw on a range of informal sources. Households are embedded in extensive and sometimes overlapping networks that can span generations, workplaces, friends, relatives and health advisors (Dew *et al.* 2014; Fainzang 2017). These networks are sources of practices for wellness that households mix together and hybridise (Latour 1993). The term health 'advisor' is used deliberately here to illustrate the notion that clinicians and specialists feed in to household strategies but by no means dictate them. Other sources come through householders' own research, using libraries and the Internet, and systematic or opportunistic reading.

## Hierarchies of advice

Unsurprisingly, the advice of health professionals finds its way into the home, but householders have to determine what health professional to trust. Medical doctors, although universally consulted by householders in our research, were not always seen as the most trustworthy of professionals. Pharmacists were frequently sought out for advice. Tania had a hierarchy of health professionals: 'If it's drugs I go straight to the pharmacist'. Zoe too articulated a hierarchy of preferred consultants that went from the health food shop, to the pharmacy, to the doctor as the last step.

Zoe's hierarchy may well be related to issues of cost: in New Zealand, consulting a health food shop assistant would be free but consulting a doctor incurs an out-of-pocket payment. But cost was by no means the only concern. Natasha was reluctant to take a remedy suggested by a friend because of her concerns that it might interfere with her medications. To resolve this, she would consult her chiropractor, who is 'probably at the top of the hierarchy – the chiropractor ... seems to know more about how systems work and how things affect each other'. For Natasha, the chiropractor would be the most expensive option – patients in New Zealand would only have chiropractic treatment subsidised if their condition was the result of an accident.

Sylvia, who has studied aromatherapy, consults 'some pretty heavy reference books' in her bedroom, and identifies networks of health professionals who use essential oils whom she consults as they are important in ensuring that she is using them in a safe way. Hazel explains why she took advice from her pharmacist about treatment for her heartburn, which was a result of taking Nurofen for period pain. Her doctor had suggested taking an additional medication to 'mask the side effects of the acid', which Hazel thought was 'a very dumb thing to do'. Hazel's nutritionist had 'more of an extreme view probably about diets and things like that and it would be a longer term approach – this really perfect diet all the time'. Instead of these extremes, she went to the pharmacist who advised omega oils, which for Hazel was a middle way. Hazel works through her health advisors until she obtains the right advice for her. We see something similar with Jim who obtains information from a range of sources that he weighs up. He rejects advice from accident and emergency staff to take medications for his rolled ankle, tries arnica and, from his reading of 'papers and stuff' he:

> [H]eard that acupuncture was very good for injuries … so that's why I went for that and again I asked around and heard someone recommend a Chinese doctor that I went to. Again, I did my own research to check he's not one of these cowboys or anything like that.

Jim's strategy evolves in dynamic fashion as he draws on different sources: health professionals, friends, alternative health practitioners, books and other reading material. Health professionals can also play a role in legitimating decisions. In regards to Anti-Flamme, a herb-based medication that Zoe uses, she says: 'I see that my physiotherapist uses it as well so that's given me a bit more confidence'. Zoe does not have so much faith in people who prescribe remedies as they may have some pecuniary interest in doing so.

## Informal sources of advice

Relatives and friends are sources of strategies. Hazel takes a zinc formula for colds that her brother suggested. She has used grapefruit seed extract – she had had 'a few funny years of poor health', and took it on the advice from a friend:

> She's a nurse, her husband's a doctor but they're also into alternative medicines themselves … If you look on the Internet, in fact, with this it's not clear. It doesn't have lots of research and there's actually websites that say, 'Don't take this stuff, it's toxic' … I do think what triggered it was my friend suggesting it.

Hazel considers different sources of information before following the advice of a friend. Her friend has what could be described as a high level of cultural health capital.

The concept of cultural health capital is derived from the work of French social theorist Pierre Bourdieu, who suggested that cultural capital was one source of power, alongside other resources such as economic capital and social capital. This source of power resided in cultural practices that could reap rewards for the individual, such as education credentials, but also things like styles of dress, food tastes and so on that could provide some distinction between those categorised as cultured (Bourdieu 1986). Janet Shim suggests that the concept of cultural health capital is important in determining the kind of interactions that occur between health professionals and others. Cultural health capital refers to the skills that we have developed or that are available to us, the sort of competency we have and our interactional styles that influence health care interactions (Shim 2010).

To return to Hazel, we can see that she is drawing on the cultural health capital of her friend. Her friend's cultural health capital is seen in her training as a health professional, a nurse, but in addition in the fact that her husband is a doctor. These characteristics carry authority for Hazel. So even though some websites paint a negative picture of her chosen remedy, grapefruit seed extract, she trusts her friend with high cultural health capital over a website that does not provide a similar sense of authority. Other householders had friends or relatives who had high levels of cultural health capital, such as homeopaths, naturopaths, osteopaths and chiropractors and the relationship of trust in them extended to trust in their expertise.

Trusted advice could come down through the generations. Tania took psyllium hulls to promote bowel motions, as suggested by her mother, who 'went totally holistic' after being diagnosed with cancer. Trust in orthodox prescriptions is transferred across generations. Hazel takes Ibuprofen when menstrual pain stops her sleeping, something her mother told her about. Similarly, Sylvia used Bonjela teething gel for her baby, recommended by her mother. In our interviews, men did not note intergenerational influences, and fathers were not identified as important in health networks. This supports a common sociological understanding of the gendered nature of care in the household, where women take on the bulk of domestic and caring work (Craig 2006).

Workplaces could act as a source of therapeutic information that comes into the household.

Jim notes that when he hears people at work talk about something that has helped them, he puts that in his 'memory bank'. Dan works at a childcare facility. The consenting systems at the facility provoked researching activities:

> In the first aid kits you have to sign for whether or not you're happy for your child to have these alternatives medicines used and, having done some research on them … [I] decided that I was happy for them to be used and later found that actually they were quite effective.

A workmate of Avril's was a yoga teacher and he 'gave me that mixture and told me to take it. It's an Ayurvedic thing'. Similarly, Louisa used a homeopathic remedy recommended by a colleague at work who was a homeopath. She was 'beside' herself as a result of frequent urinary tract infections that were not responding to specialist help from her urologist or others, but her colleague's recommendation 'worked so well that I continue to use it'. Workplaces can be both sources of information and spaces of observation, and can provoke research into wellness strategies that are subsequently deployed in the home.

It is well established that people use the Internet to access information about medications (Nettleton 2004) and for the participants in our research it was no different. The Internet can be used to access material from trusted sources and organisations, and to locate specific treatment advice. It was common for householders to use the Internet to research medications they had been prescribed, sometimes leading to the rejection of health professional advice. For example, Mark was prescribed a cholesterol-lowering medication 'and when I read up about it I don't want to take it'. Householders demonstrated an awareness of concerns about the Internet as a trusted source. Paula and Mark were impressed with what they heard on the radio about a medication for blood pressure. They checked it on the computer, but would not purchase the product until they had consulted 'the blood doctor'.

Some householders consulted books in libraries after receiving a diagnostic label, others found advice from organisations that supported people with the condition they had, and others came across recommendations in a more haphazard way, such as coming across an article in a magazine. It was rare for participants to claim influence from television. Natasha, however, suspected that she chose a particular cold sore medication because she saw it on the TV. It was more common for participants to suggest that they were not influenced by that particular source.

In sum, friends and relatives can be important sources informing wellness strategies, and the advice of health professionals is assessed for its merit and brought into the mix to determine the treatment plan in the household. We see here the Internet being used in different ways: to find good advice, to check up on prescribed medications, to follow up on information gathered elsewhere and what is found is assessed against other sources of information. Sources of advice are multiple and at times at variance with each other. Householders make sense of this, developing their own hierarchies of trust and seeking out sources that fit their own understandings and desires, using some sources to subvert recommendations from others.

Having explored how decisions are made in the household, I will now turn to some other spaces where decisions are made, to get a sense of the contrasts that occur in different contexts of health and well-being strategising.

## The contestation of pharmaceutical practices in the clinic

Chapter 8 will explore the topic of side effects in some detail, with a particular focus on how the issue of side effects is handled in the consultation between health professionals and patients. In this section we will have a look at how patients in the clinic responded to more general concerns about pharmaceuticals.

Keeping with the concepts of hybridisation and purification introduced in the previous chapter, we can see by looking at actual consultations between patients and health professionals some ways in which attempts, by both, are made to maintain 'purity' in a therapeutic approach. These endeavours are to maintain pure, unsullied categories, such as medical practice based on science, and only science. The data in this section only looks at consultations with medically trained health professionals, and not others such as naturopaths and osteopaths, but it is likely that similar purification attempts are made in their clinics as well. One way to maintain purity is to undermine or de-legitimise any challenges to expert understandings. In the case of the general practitioner (GP) clinic dis-cussed shortly, understandings drawn from non-orthodox medical knowledge are undermined. It is not that hybridising does not occur, or that categories do not get messed up. Rather, certain forms of truth production are not well accom-modated, such as ways of knowing based on the understandings of non-expert individuals, or on intuition, or on understandings arising from other therapeutic domains outside of the health professional's training (see Dew 2016, for a further discussion on the purification and hybridisation processes in different health care settings).

In the following, I will look closely at three examples of interaction between health professionals and patients that illustrate different ways in which purifica-tion efforts are made in the clinical consultation. The first two examples are from research exploring the referral processes in primary and secondary care (Dew *et al.* 2010; Dew *et al.* 2008). The third example is from research that explored issues of cancer health inequalities and health services (Dew *et al.* 2015). The first example illustrates the purified category being maintained, at least in the consultation itself; the second illustrates a compromise between categories; and the third illustrates purified categories being maintained, but in the third example the maintenance of purity, however, disrupts the consultation.

In the first example, taken from an interaction between a patient and a GP in a clinic, we see the patient make a request for a blood test, but when queried about this a problem arises when the patient suggests that he wants to follow an altern-ative diet. The patient and the doctor quickly identify the interactional problem, which is that this idea is not allowable in this space, and they both work to deal with that problem, as we will see in the transcript in Textbox 6.1. This example is from part of a consultation where the clinician is looking at the computer and talking to the patient. A brief note on the transcription convention here: I want to identify the overlaps in talk and I have done this using a convention taken from conversation analysis, where the square brackets lined up indicate that some-thing is said by both participants in the conversation at the same time.

This piece of transcript does not refer to pharmaceuticals, but I am using it here because it illustrates so nicely some of the mechanisms used to maintain purity in the clinic. I like to use this example in my teaching as it beautifully demonstrates the rapidity with which these activities of purification occur, and

---

**Textbox 6.1 Blood tests transcript**

```
 1 GP: and um now you had blood tests they were all last
 2     year
 3 PT: do you know wha- what my blood type is
 4 GP: no [I haven't] done a test for your blood type
 5 PT:    [  no  ]
 6 PT: oh okay
 7 GP: if you want me to do a test I will but there'll be small
 8     charge for that
 9 PT: yeah yep okay it's just I was thinking maybe doing a diet
10     that um- and they need you know it's good to know what your
11     blood type is and they tell you what type of food to eat
12 ((GP turns from computer and faces patient))
13 GP: oh yeah ((inhales))
14 PT: yeah or [not ]
15 GP:         [well] if you want to it I mean it there's
16     [none of these diets ]
17 PT: [nah I don't think so]
18 GP: have any great basis I have to say
19 PT: nah oh you just got to eat healthy [that's all]
20 GP:                                    [I think   ] you've just
21 got to [eat] a varied
22 PT:    [yep]
23 GP: [die-] actually the mediterranean diet's the one
24 PT: [yep ]
25 GP: we're [all] supposed to be eating
26 PT:      [yep]
27 PT: yep
28 GP: and doing a bit of exercise
29 PT: yeah yeah yeah I know
30 GP: so if you're doing [that] alan
31 PT:                    [yeah]
32 GP: [you're fine   ]
33 PT: [nah no problem]
34 GP: is that okay
35 PT: yep yep
```

---

how mundane they are. The rapidity of purification is seen most clearly on Lines 13 and 14. At this point, the patient has explained what he wants the blood tests for by making reference to an unorthodox approach to dieting known as the blood type diet, which has been disparagingly referred to as a fad diet but one that gained popularity when followed by some famous actors. By the time the clinician has processed this information, and she does this whilst she turns from the computer, says 'oh yeah' and inhales, the patient has immediately realised that something is amiss, and he goes straight to a retraction before any discussion on the matter is had, with the patient saying 'or not'.

From here on, the patient strongly affiliates with anything the clinician says, seen in the array of 'yep' and other utterances in Lines 17, 19, 22, 24, 26, 27, 29,

31, 33 and 35. The patient has completely surrendered to the GP's perspective, the strong affiliations suggesting that the patient is making every attempt to move on from the topic because he knows that he has erred. We can see from this how attuned the patient is to 'illegitimate' knowledge, how quickly positions can change, how little evidence is required when one 'legitimate' view dominates, and how little effort is made by the doctor to understand the reasons for holding 'illegitimate' views. The expert role and the purified category of what could be termed orthodoxy (purportedly based on science and rationality) are interactionally enacted. The doctor's position is not disturbed by having to consider an unorthodox view.

However, this is just what occurs in the clinical consultation. The doctor's advice may or may not be taken up outside of the clinic. The patient may have retracted his request and interactionally aligned with the expert, but once outside it is possible he will pursue his interest in fad diets by other routes. In this interaction the doctor has worked to steer the patient away from something, but has not explored why the patient was drawn to the diet in the first place, and this issue is not revisited in the consultation.

The next example examines how a contested claim is more thoroughly worked through. In this case, reasoning does occur that challenges the purified categories used by the doctor. The patient does not act passively in this example, and this leads to a compromise of sorts, at least during the consultation. In this case we can suggest, at least tentatively, that attempts to maintain purified categories of knowledge have not been successful.

---

**Textbox 6.2 Biased back transcript**

```
 1 PT: and since coming back my [back's] been a bit biased and it
 2 GP:                          [mm    ]
 3 PT: sort of yoyo's I feel its getting better but then it
 4     um like last night it's horrible finding positions to sleep
 5     [cos] the pain's going [down this leg              ]
 6 GP: [mm ]                  [the pain's going down there]
 7 GP: yeah
 8 PT: and ((exhales))
 9 GP: what can you do
10 PT: what can I do any I don't
11 GP: mm
12 PT: yeah I'm tempted to go and see my chiropractor and
13     just get a checkup
14 GP: well you could what you can do though the usual things
15     we tell you now anti-inflammatory tablets and or
16     panadol or paracetamol
17 PT: right
18 GP: and some exercises I mean you know some of the exercises to
19     do don't you and just watching your posture especially
20     with the kids cos you'll be bending down
21 ((lines omitted))
22 GP: yeah [how wo-] how would you feel about just doing your
```

```
23 PT:      [   um ]
24 GP: exercise and taking some anti inflammatory tablets jenny
25 PT: I don't like the thought of taking anti
26     inflammatories for the - it's not getting rid of the
27     problem…
  ((lines omitted))
28 GP: and allow you to do some exercises to strengthen your back
29     and to strengthen your tummy muscles again (.) and things
30     like walking going for a [swim you know go]
31 PT:                          [yeah so all    ] the things I
32     do naturally
33 GP:     yeah
34 PT: so it's [yeah      ]
35 GP:         [so you can] do that if you want to go and see
36     your chiropractor
37 PT: yeah
38 GP: you know I'll leave that to you yep
39 PT: okay I'll see how I go
```

We can see here that the patient mitigates her proposal to see her chiropractor, an activity that would mix up the purified categories of the orthodox medical consultation, as the chiropractor may hold alternative understandings of the problem with which the patient presents. The mitigation is seen in the patient stating that she is 'tempted' (Line 12), but it is clear that the activity of consulting a chiropractor is not unusual for her: she refers to 'my chiropractor', suggesting someone she has seen before and is likely to see again. The GP attempts to dissuade the patient from seeing her chiropractor by offering a contrasting approach, starting at Line 14. This approach has a focus on the use of pharmaceuticals. The patient is quite overt in not aligning with this plan, by saying 'I don't like the thought of taking anti inflammatories it's not getting rid of the problem' on Lines 25 and 26. The patient is indicating that she has a particular understanding of how back pain should be addressed, and that a chemical solution is not the one that aligns with her understanding. The patient further resists the suggestion made by her GP to supplement the use of medications with exercises by saying 'all the things I do naturally' on Lines 31 and 32. The patient is signalling that she already follows the suggestions being made and they have not resolved her complaint.

We could perhaps suggest that both parties to the conversation start off with a 'purified' position – follow the orthodox advice of the GP or pursue an alternative by attending a chiropractor. At this stage the purified positions seem to be incompatible. However, by the end of this part of the consultation there is an alignment of sorts, with the GP saying you can 'see your chiropractor' (Lines 35 and 36), so allowing for the mixing of different therapeutic approaches. The GP has acquiesced to a hybrid position in the face of persistent patient opposition. It should be noted that it is quite rare in our data set of consultations (and we have hundreds) to see such overt opposition from a patient, and this contrasts with the first example where the patient offers no resistance whatsoever. But even in this case, once the GP has shifted position, the patient shifts to possibly align with the GP's original view by stating that she will 'see how I go' (Line 39), suggesting the possibility that the mixing might not take place. All options are now available, but may or may not be pursued.

The final example from the consultation space illustrates the maintenance of purified categories, but, from a biomedical perspective, with likely negative consequences for the patient (see Dew *et al.* 2015). In this example, the patient recalls a consultation where a treatment plan was being made in response to a cancer diagnosis. The consultation was between a Māori patient and a non-Māori health practitioner. Māori are the indigenous people of New Zealand, and Māori may draw on particular therapeutic approaches that have been developed within Māori culture. The following transcript refers to rongoā, which is a Māori therapeutic approach to healing that can include spiritual healing, plant-based medicines and massage. In this transcript, excerpt from an interview with the patient, she provides an account of her response to suggestions made by the oncologist to have orthodox treatments for the cancer:

> I said, 'No, I'm not going that way. I'm going to stay with the rongoā'. The Māori herbal way. Because it was a holistic approach. And it clashed straight away … I walked out of that meeting. I ran out … I basically said, 'Get fucked to you', and left … Because I didn't like … the fact that he could sit there and pooh pooh … my way of wanting to get it fixed at that time. And basically telling me I'm a dead person if I go the rongoā way.

In this instance we see a very strong clash between different 'purified' approaches, one described as holistic by the interviewee, which is contrasted to whatever treatment she was being offered in the consultation with the oncologist. The woman perceived that the oncologist was ridiculing her approach. It is likely that the oncologist was trying to do what he thought was best for his patient, that she follow his prescribed pathway for a potentially life-threatening condition, a pathway, which would have included very toxic and powerful chemotherapy drugs and perhaps radiotherapy. For this particular oncologist there does not appear to be a way to hybridise his patient's desire with his own goals. So in this case the purified categories are reinforced, with biomedicine and rongoā medicine staying separate and unhybridised. This type of interaction may have a number of negative consequences: from a biomedical perspective the patient may not access the desired treatment; from a health care perspective the patient may have lost faith or trust in biomedicine and limit consultations with health professionals in the future.

The examples discussed provide evidence of different ways in which categories or forms of knowledge can be purified and stabilised or mixed up and undermined. There are differences between patients and practitioners in relation to what therapeutic technologies and ways of knowing are allowable. There are different means of understanding that are being accessed in these various interactions. In the case where patients table something unorthodox – a diet, a consultation with a chiropractor and the use of indigenous healing approaches – the patient may well have greater access to therapeutic systems. Patients may have acquainted themselves with what is unorthodox, and may well have more knowledge of the unorthodox than the GP. This may make it more difficult for the clinician to enact expertise in an area they know little about.

The health professional clinic is a space of intermingling, with legitimised ways of knowing being enacted as well as undermined. In the clinic, this can happen in a very finely tuned way, with patients being keenly aware of their transgressions, and in our examples either retracting and aligning with the health professional, compromising their position or withdrawing from the consultation. In the health professional consultation room, attempts are made to tame the unruly hybridised nature of everyday life. At the household level, we witness how categories that might appear fixed and stable outside the home – for example, in the clinical consultation setting – are rendered flexible and hybridised inside the home.

## The central site of the home

It is uncommon for households to provide accounts of just doing what the doctor tells them.

Householders generally construct themselves as actively participating in disputes over risks and confronting uncertainties in determining their wellness strategies. Hobson-West (2007) notes this process in relation to what she calls vaccine-critical groups, where those who question the use of vaccines on their children feel required to take on greater responsibility for their children's health and to understand complex arguments about immunisation. Householders similarly undertake this sort of work and responsibility, to varying degrees, in relation to their own therapeutic practices. The exploration of households' use of medications suggests that there is a continuum here in relation to a wide array of medication practices, in which most householders do not rely on just one source of advice.

Viewing households as hybrid centres of medication practices has implications for a sociological understanding of households and health. In terms of the sociological understanding of households, Prior has argued that we should be cautious about imputing expertise to those who have not been medically trained, as they can be wrong, and they only have their own experience or the experience of others close by to draw on. He states that patients are 'rarely skilled in matters of (medical) fact gathering, or in the business of diagnosis' (Prior 2003: 45) and are not 'skilled and practised in the diagnosis and management of illness' (Prior 2003: 53).

I am not assessing the skill levels of householders, however, householders are frequently required to make tentative diagnoses when deciding if outside health care expertise needs to be called on. In making decisions, householders gather facts and opinions from a wide range of sources. Householders are critically engaged in their therapeutic practices, that is, they reflect on and question the understandings of others and their own understandings and practices. This is not to deny that householders identify outside experts who can, and often do, play a central part in their determinations. Paul Bissell and colleagues have argued, in relation to the use of non-prescription medicines, that lay people are both experts who make choices or have agency over their decisions and are, at the same time, dependent on medicine (Bissell, Ward, and Noyce 2001). Sylvie Fainzang makes a similar point. People self-medicate making decisions, without consultation with health advisors, about what pharmaceuticals to use and when. So in that sense they can act independently of medical practitioners. But this is also a process of self-medicalisation, in that, in her study, lay people define the problem in medical language (Fainzang 2017).

Stuart McClean and Alison Shaw demonstrate, in relation to food risks and alternative medicine use, that lay people 'adopt, mimic, critique, or rewrite expert positions' (McClean and Shaw 2005: 746). This adopting and rewriting occurs not only in relation to experts, but in relation to friends, relatives, colleagues and a range of search activities. However, we should note a limitation here, in that our research did not focus on acute conditions, which likely shift the focus of trust onto a narrower range of influences. That is, when we are in intense pain or have some other dramatic and activity-limiting symptoms, we are likely to go to the sources that provide opportunities for quick remedies, and for many people that will involve falling back on medically trained personnel and a likelihood of taking prescribed medications. One of our householders explicitly references this: Janice stated that she preferred naturopathic products to treat problems, but 'I suppose if I got cancer I would go straight to the allopathic stuff' (Chamberlain *et al.* 2011: 304). Thus, householders may draw on different forms of governance depending upon the particular situation.

I suggest that households are a central site of health practices and decision-making. Historians have claimed that home health practices became severely restricted and less common with the rise in dominance of the medical profession (Risse 1993; Wear 1995). In seventeenth century England, 'Well-stocked homes had kitchen-physic: bottles of homebrewed or shop-bought purges, vomits, pain-killers, cordials, febrifuges (medicines to reduce fever) and the like', and people were 'less doctor dependent than today' (Porter 1987: 29). Anthropologists have shown how home health practices are predominant in non-western cultures where the purchase of 'professional biomedicine' is limited, implying a lack of home health practices in the West (Waldstein 2010). Sociologists have argued that in recent times, a new medical cosmology has developed as a consequence of medical knowledge becoming unbound from medical institutions through new technologies, primarily through the use of the Internet (Nettleton 2004). More ready access to medical knowledge opens up the possibility of more home-based health practices. I am arguing that the disappearance of therapeutic practices from the home in the West may have been overstated. Professional biomedicine does have a purchase on the home in contemporary times, but the practices of professional biomedicine are thoroughly mixed with other wellness strategies and reworked in the home. Although the Internet can be a source of wellness strategies, there are and always have been, many other sources going across generations, workplaces and through social networks as well as technological networks. By looking at the wellness strategies in the home it can be argued that medical knowledge has never been successfully bound up in medical institutions or professional biomedicine. Medical practitioners and other health providers have always been but one source of strategies.

This view of households, as the space where decisions are made based on outside advice, experimentation and observation, has consequences for health practitioners. For example, the meaningfulness of the goal of 'concordance' in medical decision-making, which became a prominent feature of consultation discussions in the 1990s (Mead and Bower 2000), is questioned as a result of gaining a better understanding of household health practices. Concordance has been defined as:

> An agreement reached after negotiation between a patient and a healthcare professional that respects the beliefs and wishes of the patient in determining whether, when, and how medicines are to be taken.
>
> (Dickinson, Wilkie, and Harris 1999)

Such a notion has an underlying assumption of the patient as individualised, and decision-making as a static event that occurs once in a consulting room, as opposed to decision-making being dynamic and embedded within a networked collective, the medical doctor being but one (although very often a crucially important) node in the network. Considering the home as a health practice in its own right challenges the centrality of the medical consultation in medication practices and directs us to the everyday and collective nature of health care decision-making.

## Concluding comments

Over the last three chapters, I have discussed in some detail everyday understandings and practices about health treatments. The use of the concept of hybridity provides a focus that questions the compartmentalising of categories into orthodox and alternative, artificial and natural. These categories are intertwined and mixed in health maintenance activities in the household. The term 'hybrid' supports the image of households as nodes in complex networks of advice, practice and expertise. Drawing on de Certeau, it is argued here that households are active producers of medication practices, using but manipulating frameworks drawn from outside the household. This manipulation and production of practices applies as much to the frameworks of alternative practitioners as it does to the frameworks of orthodox medicine.

Householders necessarily develop expertise in wellness strategies through experimentation, research activities and consultations with numerous advisors and acquaintances. They draw on their own hierarchies of trust; they use health advisors as tools for developing their own medication practices and wellness strategies; and, householders subvert normative frameworks and evade being disciplined by the practices encountered in the consultation rooms of health practitioners. Subversion can be seen in processes of rejecting, modifying and tactically forgetting clinical advice and recommendations. Personal medication practices develop from practical concerns over medication use, resource issues and congruence with worldviews, and through processes of experimentation and observation. We can thus, usefully conceptualise the household as the centre of a networked therapeutic practice that actively hybridises therapeutic advice.

Chapter 3 provided a sense of the inexorable processes of medicalisation that would appear to draw us all in to increasingly constrained forms of pharmaceuticalised governance. The last three chapters indicate how processes of medicalisation, pharmaceuticalisation and biomedicalisation manifest in the home. We see how forms of pharmaceuticalised governance are resisted. We also see how householders engage in their own forms of pharmaceuticalised governance by consuming medications and combining therapeutic practices in unanticipated ways, not overseen by the state or the health professional. Governance in relation to health care takes many forms. The following chapter shifts the focus to consider ways in which concerns around population health provide some very powerful levers to enhance pharmaceuticalised governance and challenge the autonomy of the householder.

## Appendix

The following are the transcription conventions used in some of the transcripts.

| | |
|---|---|
| (.) | denotes a micro-pause |
| (2) | denotes a pause of the specified number of seconds |
| [ ] | denotes overlapping talk |
| (and) | words in single parentheses denote candidate hearings |
| <u>Certainly</u> | underlined word denotes increased emphasis |
| = | denotes latching or no gap between talk |
| ((laughs)) | words in double parentheses denotes descriptions that have been added by the author |
| GP: | refers to the general practitioner speaking |
| PT: | refers to the patient speaking |

## References

Bissell, P., Ward, P. and Noyce, P. (2001). The dependent consumer: Reflections on accounts of the risks of non-prescription medicines. *Health* 5 (1): 5–30.

Bourdieu, P. (1986). The forms of capital. In: *Handbook of Theory of Research for the Sociology of Education* (ed. J. Richardson), 241–258). New York: Greenwood Press.

Chamberlain, K., Madden, H., Gabe, J., Dew, K. and Norris, P. (2011). Forms of resistance to medication within New Zealand households. *Medische Anthroplogie* 23 (2): 299–308.

Craig, L. (2006). Children and the revolution: A time-diary analysis of the impact of motherhood on daily workload. *Journal of Sociology* 42 (2): 124–144.

Dew, K. (2016). Purifying and hybridising categories in healthcare decision-making: The clinic, the home and the multidisciplinary team. *Health Sociology Review* 25 (2): 142–156.

Dew, K., Chamberlain, K., Hodgetts, D., Norris, P., Radley, A. and Gabe, J. (2014). Home as a hybrid centre of medication practice. *Sociology of Health and Illness* 36 (1): 28–43.

Dew, K., Plumridge, E., Stubbe, M., Dowell, A., Macdonald, L. and Major, G. (2008). 'You just got to eat healthy': The topic of CAM in the general practice consultation. *Health Sociology Review* 17 (4): 396–409.

Dew, K., Signal, L., Davies, C., Tavite, H., Hooper, C., Safati, D., Stairmand, J. and Cunningham, C. (2015). Dissonant roles: The experience of Māori in cancer care. *Social Science and Medicine* 138: 144–151.

Dew, K., Stubbe, M., Macdonald, L., Dowell, A. and Plumridge, E. (2010). The (non)use of prioritisation protocols by surgeons. *Sociology of Health and Illness* 32 (4): 545–562.

Dickinson, D., Wilkie, P. and Harris, M. (1999). Taking medicines: Concordance is not compliance. *British Medical Journal* 319: 787.

Fainzang, S. (2017). *Self-Medication and Society: Mirages of Autonomy.* Abingdon: Routledge.

Hobson-West, P. (2007). 'Trusting blindly can be the biggest risk of all': Organised resistance to childhood vaccination in the UK. *Sociology of Health and Illness* 29 (2): 198–215.

McClean, S. and Shaw, A. (2005). From schism to continuum? The problematic relationship between expert and lay knowledge – An exploratory conceptual synthesis of two qualitative studies. *Qualitative Health Research* 15 (6): 729–749. doi: 10.1177/1049 732304273927.

Mead, N. and Bower, P. (2000). Patient-centredness: A conceptual framework and review of the empirical literature. *Social Science and Medicine* 51: 1087–1110.

Nettleton, S. (2004). The emergence of e-scaped medicine? *Sociology* 38 (4): 661–679.

Porter, R. (1987). *Disease, Medicine and Society in England 1550–1860.* Basingstoke: Macmillan.

Prior, L. (2003). Belief, knowledge and expertise: The emergence of the lay expert in medical sociology. *Sociology of Health and Illness* 25: 41–57.

Risse, G. (1993). Medical care. In: *Companion Encyclopedia of the History of Medicine* (eds W.F. Bynum and R. Porter), 45–77. London and New York: Routledge.

Shim, J. (2010). Cultural health capital: A theoretical approach to understanding health care interactions and the dynamics of unequal treatment. *Journal of Health and Social Behavior* 51 (1): 1–15.

Waldstein, A. (2010). Popular medicine and self-care in a Mexican migrant community: Toward an explanation of an epidemiological paradox. *Medical Anthropology* 29 (1): 71–107.

Wear, A. (1995). Medicine in early modern Europe, 1500–1700. In: *The Western Medical Tradition: 800 BC to AD 1800* (ed. L.I. Conrad), 215–361. Cambridge: Cambridge University Press.

# 7  Populations and medications

In this chapter, the technology of vaccination is discussed to consider the ways in which powerful public health narratives and mechanisms can intensify pharmaceuticalised governance. For some, devoting a chapter to vaccines in a book primarily focused on the influence of pharmaceuticals on our conduct may seem out of place, but it is here for a particular purpose. Vaccines stand out as one of the great hopes of medical practice, as a signifier of the power of medical interventions, as much as, if not more than, antibiotics (or than antibiotics did – if the concern about a post-antibiotic era are borne out). Vaccines are such a powerful signifier because they are viewed as a means of disease eradication – smallpox being the classic example. The hope is that if the world can eliminate the deadly disease of smallpox, it may be able to eliminate all infectious diseases. Vaccines are seen as the reason for low levels of infectious diseases in many developed countries, diseases that wreaked havoc in the nineteenth and twentieth centuries, such as measles, whooping cough and poliomyelitis.

But the power of vaccines is also a concern. The goal of preventing infectious diseases in populations is a noble one, but sometimes the means of achieving that end is not so noble. The use of, at times, unsavoury means by those responsible for vaccination development, policy and delivery is rarely acknowledged, and it certainly was not something I was aware of when I embarked on my forays into a sociology of vaccination. My gradual awakening to a critique of some aspects of vaccination policy is not unique, and with a little research one can find a literature related to vaccine critique and resistance. A comparison between vaccines and pharmaceuticals is informative, both in the different ways they are understood and in the discourse of shared responsibility for health that is central to vaccination policies and may become more central to pharmaceuticals.

The very act of writing this chapter will be received by some as anti-vaccination pseudo-science, or as a dangerous approach to take because it might influence vulnerable and irrational people to take anti-vaccination positions. It is not my goal at all to promote an anti-vaccination stance, but I have come to the position that we have a duty to consistently interrogate both vaccination policy and the means taken to facilitate high levels of vaccine coverage.

My position is not a stable and unchanging one. Before I undertook any research on vaccinations, I accepted the standard medical story of vaccines and passively submitted myself to the technology. In the literature, this position has been referred to as being an 'acceptor', where I was simply relying on social norms (Brunson 2013). My own personal experience of vaccines was not particularly problematic. On vaccination day at school we were all lined up and the needles went into our arms in very quick fashion. Needle-phobia had a dramatic impact upon some, but only elicited standard nervousness on my part. On another occasion, when my family was about to embark overseas for a number of years, we were all given a cocktail of vaccines for, to me, exotic diseases like yellow fever. I was fine with these vaccines, but my sister and my mother had days of illness following the doctor's visit. To me this was simply a minor cost of a necessary procedure.

I did not really think about vaccines again until many years later when I was studying osteopathy. In some of the older osteopathic writings there were arguments made against the use of vaccines, but to me these seemed distant and historic pieces of writing – much had happened in medical science since those days. However, a student in a class below me came to me one day and asked me about vaccination issues. His wife was just about to have their first child and he was a little unsure about vaccinations; he wanted to know if I had any useful information on this from an osteopathic perspective. I knew of nothing, but at around about that time I came across a book called *Vaccination and Immunisation: Delusions and Alternatives* by Leon Chaitow (1987), a British trained naturopath and osteopath. This was the first extended text I had read that took a critical perspective on vaccinations, and Chaitow provided many examples of controversies, disputes and debates about this technology that were unknown to me.

My next encounter with the vaccination issue came many years later when I had returned to New Zealand to complete an honours degree in sociology. As part of the honours programme I undertook a research project, and I chose to focus on media coverage of measles epidemics. I did so because, as I was preparing for honours, a measles epidemic was occurring and I was quite surprised by the newspaper coverage of the epidemic. My interest was initially piqued because when I was a child, measles was an illness that children were expected to get. When I and my siblings had measles we were not even taken to the doctor as it was such a common experience that it was dealt with in the home.

My own personal experience is reflected in the medical literature of the time. In 1962, Langmuir and his colleagues of the epidemiology branch of the Communicable Disease Center of the United States (US) Public Health Service argued that measles should be eradicated, not because of concerns about the disability and morbidity that it caused in the US, but because the tools for eradication were becoming available and, quoting the answer given by my compatriot Edmund Hillary on why he wanted to climb Everest, 'because it is there' (Langmuir *et al.* 1962). From an epidemiological perspective, the disease was not a concern in affluent countries, although it was, and still is, a concern in countries where people are malnourished and poor. But the newspaper coverage I saw seemed to promise disaster of plague proportions if the epidemic was not contained. As a research project, I decided to make comparisons of newspaper coverage during different epidemics, first just to see if the coverage had increased over time, but in addition to see if anything else was different about the coverage (for a detailed discussion of my findings see Dew 1999). A few events occurred during this research that had quite a profound effect upon me.

The first event was coming to the realisation that I had in all likelihood been a recipient of a contaminated vaccine. In undertaking the research project I tried to read all I could about the history of vaccine usage in New Zealand. In doing so, I discovered that in the 1960s a polio vaccine known to be contaminated with the monkey virus SV40 (simian virus 40) was knowingly administered to millions of people in a number of countries (Martin 1996), including New Zealand. Polio vaccines were cultured in the live kidneys of monkeys, making possible the contamination of such vaccines with unknown viruses that remained invisible as they may have had no deleterious effect on their natural monkey hosts. The risks of such a procedure and the SV40 example has led a number of researchers to suggest that contaminated polio vaccines, which were administered in mass immunisation programmes in West and Central Africa, are the origin of the AIDS pandemic (Martin 1996). In New Zealand the health department took the view that the public did not need to know about the contamination, and even prevented a virologist wanting to investigate the issue from accessing the relevant files (Day 2008).

This discovery that contaminated vaccines had been deliberately used gave me pause for thought. Health authorities had made the decision to use the contaminated vaccines without informing parents and the public. Information had been controlled so that people were more likely to conform to what the 'experts' wanted. This decision could have consequences for me personally. The political was personal. I was a little shocked at the time.

The second event was an outcome of further data collection for the research project. As part of the research I conducted two purposive interviews to represent the two sides of the vaccination debate. One was with a member of the Immunisation Awareness Society (IAS), an organisation established in 1988 with the goal of getting parents to look at both sides of the immunisation debate before making a decision about vaccinating their children (introduced in an introductory anecdote in Chapter 4). The other interview was conducted with a senior medical officer from the then Department of Health. The purpose of these interviews was to look at the personal background and engagement with vaccination debates of the interviewees; to establish the reasons for their position; to ascertain what future scenarios they envisaged for measles vaccinations and their effects; and to find out their views on how the media handles these issues. Following the interviews, transcripts were sent to the two respondents and they were given the opportunity to withdraw any information they wished. The IAS respondent requested that the views she expressed be shown as her personal views and not representative of the views of anyone else, particularly the IAS. In addition she requested that some personal information be excluded. The Department of Health respondent sent back the transcript completely re-typed with an accompanying letter stating that 'I have altered the transcript substantially in order to make the points we discussed clearer'. When I offered my participants the chance to withdraw information I had not anticipated the possibility of someone taking the material and rewriting it. In this case the transcript now seemed to be more like a health information pamphlet, as opposed to an interview where beliefs, values and assumptions could be clearly discerned. It seemed to me unfair that one participant had empowered themselves in this way whilst the other did not.

Additionally, at the completion of the interview with the medical officer, after the tape was turned off, I was told in no uncertain terms that my task here was an important one and that I must tell the 'right' story in my research: the Department of Health's story. When I walked back to university after that interview I seriously considered stopping the research and changing my research topic. I had been confronted by someone who spends his working life trying to improve vaccination rates in New Zealand. It was already clear to me that the health authorities used strategies that were not always aimed at informing people, but that could rather limit debate and discussion. My developing critique would suggest that we should be wary of such efforts, but who was I to make this critique? A lowly honours student whose work might play a small part in undermining the great work of the health authorities. But soon I got angry and concluded that I was being manipulated here, and in fact it was the duty of a researcher to present his or her understanding to the world, to contribute to debate. Even if I might be wrong in some way, it was important that I took the view that a dialogue or a conversation should be encouraged.

In sum, after this initial research I started to shift my position from a passive compliant acceptor of vaccination policy to being surprised by distortions and misinformation that, at times, accompanied the standard medical story. I had become more of what Brunson (2013) calls a 'searcher', seeking out information from a range of sources to make sense of vaccination policies. I am still dismayed at some of the tactics of pro-vaccinators (see Martin 2013), but would now say that I want to promote debate, expose the suppression of dissenting voices, make values explicit, and ask whether we should leave decisions about something as important as vaccination policy in the hands of a few immunologists. So my position has changed as a result of my investigations, and may well change again.

The trajectory of my relationship to vaccines that I have just outlined is expressed in the literature exploring vaccine resistance. A study of vaccine dissent in France and Portugal found that most 'dissenters' did not start from anything like an anti-vaccination position, and do not end up in a static anti-vaccination position. Rather, dissent is something that they arrive at, as political subjects, after questioning themselves about vaccines, finding that health care institutions resisted their questions, and them seeking out those who might be more receptive to a questioning stance. That is, dissenters take on a more active relationship to bureaucratic institutions and expert systems, resisting 'overbearing state regulatory power' (Cunha and Durand 2013: 50).

Terra Manca's research on the anxieties of physicians and nurses in Canada about vaccinations further complicates the idea that to question vaccines is about as reasonable as believing the earth is flat. Research has shown that health professionals refuse to take certain vaccines themselves, with vaccination uptake for some vaccines being as low as 51 per cent. (Manca 2018). In particular, some health professionals were concerned about the efficacy and safety of newer vaccines heavily promoted by pharmaceutical companies, with particular scepticism about influenza vaccines. Others noted the occurrence of adverse reactions to vaccines, some severe, that were not part of the public health vaccine narrative. Some health professionals were concerned that patients only had partial information on which to base their decisions (Manca 2018). The concerns of health professionals do not, however, get translated into the public health narrative about vaccines.

How does this relate to pharmaceuticals and pharmaceuticalised governance? One of the major differences between vaccines and standard medications is that many, although not all, vaccines are thought to establish 'herd immunity'. Herd immunity is a powerful concept that promotes attempts to obtain universal, or near universal, population coverage of vaccines (Hobson-West 2007). Herd immunity is achieved if a high enough proportion of a population is vaccinated and if a sufficient number of individuals gain immunity to the target infectious disease from the vaccination procedure. If this occurs, then any potential reservoir for the disease is abolished; the disease can therefore be eradicated. Consequently, even those very few individuals who refuse to receive vaccinations or who get missed in vaccination campaigns will be protected. It is argued that if a significant proportion of the population is not vaccinated, then there will be a sufficient number of unvaccinated individuals susceptible to the disease, which can then become the source of an epidemic at any time. Thus, if herd immunity is not achieved, the disease cannot be eliminated, as only those specific individuals who have been vaccinated will be protected; those who have not will form a reservoir for the disease-causing agents. Given that vaccines are not 100 per cent effective in conferring immunity, even some vaccinated individuals will not be protected.

Herd immunity promotes particular forms of state or health authority governance: the concept of herd immunity supports endeavours to enforce compliance and remove the choice of whether to partake in preventive interventions or not. As another aside, at the time of writing, there is a mumps epidemic in New Zealand that has been getting a lot of coverage. This epidemic is occurring in an age group where most would have been exposed to the mumps vaccine. Commentators are suggesting that the vaccine protection wanes over time, hence the unexpected epidemic and a lack of herd immunity.

Currently, other products of pharmaceutical companies do not claim to confer herd immunity. However, there are other kinds of collective issues that may increasingly come to the fore with regards to pharmaceuticals, shifting the balance from pharmaceutical consumption being a decision that primarily impacts upon the individual to one where the community or the public might wish to have a greater say. One obvious way for this to occur is if an individual's right to choose is seen as having a negative impact on health resource use, in that 'preventive' measures now may save costs of more expensive interventions at a later time. I will draw this argument out more in the concluding chapter of this book. Another feature of vaccinations is that, as with pharmaceuticals, there are consistent attempts to expand the market. For vaccines, this means moving beyond infectious diseases to target other conditions such as cancer, chronic illness and contraception (Cunha and Durand 2013). In these developments there is perhaps something of a convergence in the trajectories of vaccinations and other medications.

## Public health and infectious diseases

The practice of vaccination to confer immunity or protection from infectious disease is held in such high regard that it is presented as a cornerstone of preventive medicine (Streefland 2001). The practice of vaccination itself can be problematic, and some concerns about it are discussed in this section, including the coercive nature of campaigns, the increasing number of vaccines being added to vaccine schedules and the overstating of claims about the impact of vaccines. The concept of biopower may help us to comprehend the development and use of vaccinations, and help us understand other pharmaceutical interventions aimed at a population level.

The exemplar and first widely used vaccine was the smallpox vaccine, which is commonly considered to have eradicated the disease worldwide. Today there are a variety of vaccines, many of which are incorporated into vaccination programmes for children. In some jurisdictions these are mandatory, whilst in others they are supported by strong coercive campaigns to increase the uptake of vaccination (Delamater *et al.* 2016; Dew 1999). An example of increasing coercive approaches to vaccine uptake can be seen in a recent social welfare policy change in Australia known as *No Jab No Pay*, in which parents of children who are unvaccinated or only partially vaccinated are ineligible for welfare payments known as Family Assistance Payments unless they have a medical exemption (Leask and Danchin 2017). New vaccines are added to national vaccine schedules on a regular basis, so in addition to the core vaccines for mumps, measles, rubella, diphtheria, poliomyelitis and tetanus, others have been added such as varicella, Haemophilus influenzae type B and meningococcal meningitis. From a public health perspective, vaccinations are a good use of resources, based on the calculations made relating the costs of the intervention to the perceived public health benefits that are conferred.

As noted, in the late nineteenth and early twentieth centuries some diseases, such as measles, scarlet fever, diphtheria, whooping cough and tuberculosis, caused many deaths in the Western world, but there was an impressive drop in mortality from these diseases from the early twentieth century. It is often assumed that this drop was the result of vaccination programmes, and the fall in death rates from infectious diseases can be seen as an outstanding success in public health. However, the role that medical intervention played in this decline has been contested, most famously by Thomas McKeown, a physician and historian, in his book *The Role of Medicine* published in 1979. McKeown (1979) argued that it was improved diet and a rising standard of living that were responsible for enhancing resistance to infectious diseases. These structural changes were responsible for the lowering of death rates, which included diseases for which there was no available vaccine such as scarlet fever. The only real exceptions here, McKeown argued, are vaccinations for smallpox and sanitary improvements reducing the impact of diseases such as cholera and typhoid (Hardy 2001). What accounted for the decline in other diseases, like scarlet fever and diphtheria, is not absolutely clear, but besides changes in sanitation and sewerage measures, nutritional changes, social changes such as education and public housing, improvements in the health of children and changes in the virulence of the disease, have all been suggested. McKeown's argument that medical measures only played a limited role in mortality decline prior to the mid-twentieth century has been accepted by demographers and historians as correct (Colgrove 2002: 728). This is not, however, the view commonly expressed by representatives of medicine and public health during outbreaks of these infectious diseases, where calls are often made that vaccination rates need to be kept up to avoid the epidemics of a century ago.

I suggest that one way of making sense of the intense focus on interventions like vaccinations is by drawing on concepts developed by French theorist Michel Foucault. Foucault argued that an increasing emphasis, by the state and its institutions, on the biological processes of the body has changed how the individual is produced as a subject that can be understood and managed (Foucault 1978). Foucault's use of the word 'subject' has a number of connotations, including a reference to the sense of self we have (as in, a subjective understanding is an understanding that is internal to me, as opposed to an objective understanding that comes from some external, and often measurable, process) and a reference to the idea that we are 'subjected' to something else (as in, the King and his subjects). Foucault argued that bodies are understood, and therefore managed, in terms of what is known about their biological composition and physiology. As noted in Chapter 3, Foucault referred to this interlinking of knowledge or understanding and biological processes as biopower. Foucault argued that we can see biopower at play in increasing concerns, by the state and by populations, over birth, mortality and longevity as indicators of the health of individuals and populations. A range of institutions take on the role of enhancing concerns with health, both state, or public and private institutions. Biological processes have become regulated through a series of interventions and controls, such as the implementation of vaccine policy, but also through many other means like developments in health screening, the use of genetic information and so on. For Foucault, the goal of taking care of the population strengthens the state (Foucault 1988).

From a Foucauldian perspective we are produced, moulded and restricted by the technologies and knowledge used to improve our health. In the name of health, means have been developed to increasingly discipline our lives from birth to death. From the needle-prick screening when a baby is born to our hospitalised deaths, we are described, prescribed and regulated. But it is not simply that these 'regimes of power' (Foucault 1984: 149) are imposed upon us. We impose them upon ourselves, and even demand them.

For Foucault, people's lives can be managed and knowledge can be collected via systems of surveillance and the normalisation of bodies. Normalisation refers to the attempt to make sick or deviant bodies comply with norms of what the body should be and how it should act. It also refers to the process of subjecting the population to standard procedures, such as mass screening and vaccinations, efforts to standardise bodies. This expression of governmentality allows for greater control or administration of bodies. By subjecting everyone to the same procedures, it becomes easier to identify those who do not conform, and therefore to develop strategies to coerce or force people to comply with the objectives of public health.

The idea of standardising bodies was touched on in Chapter 1 where it was noted that, through processes of standardising, certain groups, particularly the state, can gain greater control (Porter 1995; Scott 1998). The processes of standardisation occur in many social spaces. Researchers need to standardise their experiments so results can be reasonably compared. Not only does this mean having standardised measures, but it additionally means having comparable biological specimens for example – so there are efforts to 'standardise' biology, or to put this more dramatically, standardise life.

So how might the trends of standardisation relate to vaccines, pharmaceuticals and pharmaceuticalised governance? One way we can see this is that vaccines are an attempt to standardise the immune systems of entire populations, therefore, everyone can be treated the same in relation to infectious diseases and their prevention. This potentially makes things easier for health authorities, as they would have fewer concerns about infectious diseases if everyone had a standard response to their presence.

In relation to pharmaceuticals, there has been great attention paid to standardising the biology of bodies, and to use pharmaceuticals to gain conformity to the desired standard. We see this with cholesterol, blood pressure, glucose levels and many other measures as noted in Chapter 3. This is great news for drug companies, particularly if they can increasingly lower the threshold at which their drugs should be used (see Chapter 3 for a fuller discussion of this). A chain of logic is established: where biological processes are abnormal, and if they continue at this abnormal level there will be an increase in the chances of future disease and ill health (such as heart disease, kidney failure, diabetes), and there are drugs that can bring these biological processes back to normal, then those drugs should be used. Bodies are therefore to be standardised to reduce the future burden of disease, just as is the case with vaccines.

As noted, the concept of herd immunity provides a very powerful imperative for everyone to vaccinate. The moral imperative is one of social solidarity – if you do not vaccinate, you are being irresponsible and letting the community down. You are being a free rider: whilst other people expose themselves to the risk of adverse effects from vaccines in order to protect both themselves and the population, the non-vaccinator stands apart as morally inferior in that they are not doing their bit for the community. With pharmaceuticals, there is no concern about herd immunity. However, I would suggest that we will increasingly see powerful rhetorical strategies, based on the moral imperatives of social solidarity, developed to stigmatise those who might refuse to standardise their bodies with pharmaceuticals. One very likely strand of rhetoric will be to position those who resist preventive medications as being a future economic and social burden on society, particularly in relation to the use of scarce health resources like hospital beds and more invasive medical interventions like surgery. Today we often hear concerns raised about providing health resources to smokers or others who make poor lifestyle 'choices' (Wigginton *et al.* 2017). Should they have the same access to health resources as those who have avoided bad lifestyle 'choices'? The stigma faced by non-vaccinators, and smokers, may well be faced by those who do not comply with the prescription of preventive, standardising pharmaceuticals.

## Resisting social solidarity and the price of dissent

Although vaccines have been broadly embraced, there has been resistance to them from time-to-time. Reasons for resistance are diverse, and include concerns about adverse reactions, that vaccines may weaken the immune system, that vaccine efficacy is misrepresented, and that vaccines are a form of political tyranny.

One common concern of those few who dissent is possible adverse reactions to a vaccine. For example, with the introduction of Gardasil, a vaccine to prevent cervical cancer, a US organisation called Judicial Watch disseminated information about the number of adverse reactions to the vaccine reported to the Vaccine Adverse Event Report System. The vaccine was given to girls aged 9 and over and, as Judicial Watch pointed out, the Reporting System had collected over 3000 reported adverse events, including 11 deaths in 2007 (Nelson and Moser 2008). There has been concern, expressed more forcefully at some times than others, about the risk of combining different vaccines, seen dramatically in the controversy over the safety of the measles, mumps and rubella (MMR) vaccine discussed on page 100 (Poltorak. M. *et al.* 2005). The early age at which vaccines are given has been of concern to parents, and for some people, vaccines are viewed as potentially weakening the immune system (Cunha and Durand 2013). Another concern is the misrepresentation of so-called vaccine preventable diseases. For example, editors of medical journals have accused vaccine manufacturers of exaggerating the number of deaths that result from the absence of relevant vaccines. Authors based at the Center for Disease Control in Atlanta, US, admitted a 50-fold inflation of hepatitis B mortality in India (Puliyel and Madhavi 2008). There is, then, often considerable debate around the merits of vaccines, implementation programmes and potential adverse reactions.

Moreover, the history of vaccines has been misrepresented. So, for example, although Edward Jenner, the physician known as the developer of the smallpox vaccine, is often depicted as a hero of medicine and public health, what is not usually depicted are the likely negative consequences of his processes. Jenner's procedure, which he developed in 1772, was to inject the person to be vaccinated with pus taken from the blisters of someone who had been exposed to cowpox (Halliday 2007). At this time there was no sophisticated blood screening, and there was little knowledge of what was happening within the body as pus from pustules was forced into the blood stream. One consequence of this procedure was that other diseases were being spread through the population. Vaccines increased the risk of spreading hepatitis, leprosy and syphilis. These adverse consequences were not recognised at that time, as the accepted belief at that time was that an individual could only have one disease at a time; if someone had smallpox, they could not have any other disease (Copp and Zanella 1992).

In the early days of vaccination, vaccines were interpreted by some as a violation of the body and a form of political tyranny (Durbach 2000). The tyranny of vaccination policy can be seen in the case of a man called Jones, a detailed account of which is provided by historian Logie Barrow (2002). In 1871, in Islington, London, Jones was sent to prison for failing to present his child to a vaccination station (Barrow 2002). The compulsory vaccination laws of the time meant that Jones was required to bring his child to a vaccination station for the poor, to receive lymph vaccinations from another child. The compulsory vaccination laws made it mandatory for selected children to return a week later, to check if the vaccination had worked and to determine whether a child should be a vaccinifer – a child whose lymph would be used to vaccinate other children presenting that day. Jones was told by a medical officer not to present his child for this second surveillance visit, as there was a child dying of smallpox in his house, making him and his children at risk of spreading the disease to others. The vaccinator took the case against Jones, because Jones' child was the only potential vaccinifer for that week, and so was the only one that could provide the lymph for the arm-to-arm vaccination process (Barrow 2002). It is not surprising that in many jurisdictions there was little uptake of these regulations, as the medical profession itself did not always support and enforce them. An anti-vaccination response can therefore be seen, in this sort of situation, as a rational response to poorly administered and draconian laws.

Misrepresentations of vaccines can have unintended consequences. Mothers, who are told that immunisations do not cause any side effects, may stop further vaccination of their children after seeing side effects, such as allergic reactions, develop in one child (New and Senior 1991). In other instances, mothers stopped vaccinating their children after initial vaccines failed to protect their children from the targeted infectious disease. These responses to vaccines are examples of householders making sense of advice and treatments in relation to their own observations. Resistance to social solidarity can then come about as a result of observations of mothers or carers that lead to a questioning of vaccination procedures.

One consequence of resisting public health messages and the advice of experts is that responsibility for decision-making becomes much more personal. In her article, titled: *Trusting Blindly Can Be the Biggest Risk of All*, Pru

Hobson-West argues that those who are 'vaccine critical' put a great deal of energy into being informed and taking responsibility. To do so means not simply trusting official sources of information, but critiquing that information. It is much easier to be ignorant and to trust, because you do not have to try to follow complex arguments and you do not have to take responsibility – you can relinquish such decisions to others. Trusting in experts is, in many ways, the easier option. But for those who develop a vaccine-critical stance, such trust is itself a source of risk as experts may misinform (Hobson-West 2007).

In some states, resisting population health procedures can come at a personal and financial cost. This became apparent to me when I was made aware of the activities of a pro-vaccination citizen's group in Australia. Brian Martin from the University of Wollongong writes about his involvement in this process, noting the vitriolic response he received as a consequence of writing about attacks on a vaccine-critical group (Martin 2016). Martin says he does not have a strong view about the issue of vaccinations, his intervention deriving instead from his value commitment to freedom of speech. He notes how in 2009 a pro-vaccination group was set up to explicitly close down a vaccine-critical group in Australia, which in so doing deployed various tactics that one might expect to see in efforts to suppress dissenting views, such as personalised attacks, undermining the capacity of people to speak in public and so on. When Martin got involved by writing articles about these attacks, he too was turned on by the pro-vaccination group, not because he supported the vaccine-critical view, but because he provided information that could help the vaccine-critical group to understand the sort of attack they were under. Martin himself became the target of attacks including abusive online commentary and complaints to his university.

One of his PhD students, Judy Wilyman, was similarly subjected to attacks. Her thesis raised concerns about gaps in the scientific knowledge that underpinned vaccination policies in Australia (Wilyman 2015). Two days after her thesis was posted online, it was denigrated on the front page of a prominent Australian newspaper and was the subject of hostile articles, tweets, blogs and a petition. Her thesis prompted a commentary by two prominent public health advocates published in the journal *Vaccine*, arguing for restriction on academic freedom for research with the potential to harm human health (Durrheim and Jones 2016). Researchers need to have a very thick skin to endure attempts to suppress their work, and it would be much easier to choose topics that are not so likely to attract such negativity.

In the clinical research field, the costs of dissenting views can be more dramatic. Andrew Wakefield had a paper accepted and published in *The Lancet* in 1998, in which he and his colleagues claimed that they had found an association between the MMR vaccine and autism. The research was on too small a sample to go much further, and the article did not claim that the MMR caused autism. However, following the publication of the article, Wakefield did suggest to the media that parents should be offered the chance to have single vaccines, rather than the combined MMR vaccine, until the possible link between the vaccine and autism was further studied (Holton *et al.* 2012). This might appear to be a sound suggestion based on something like the precautionary principle, but following this, not only was Wakefield vilified as being dishonest and irresponsible, he had his paper formally retracted from the journal 12 years later, and was banned from practising as a doctor in the United Kingdom after his research was deemed by the medical council to be fraudulent. On receipt of the news of his ban, Wakefield stated that:

> It seemed to me that they had come to this decision a long time ago, long before the evidence was fairly heard. This is the way the system deals with dissent. You isolate, discredit and provide an example to other doctors and scientists not to get involved in this kind of thing. That is, examining questions of vaccine safety.
>
> (Boseley 2010)

This vilification has not stopped researchers outside of the medical field itself from studying the relationship between MMR and autism. Gayle DeLong, safely based in a Department of Economics and Finance, and therefore somewhat at arms-length from the medical world, concluded that there was a positive and statistically significant relationship between vaccination rates and autism – a higher vaccination rate was associated with a higher prevalence of autism (DeLong 2011). Not surprisingly, this finding has been subject to much criticism, but as DeLong is not a registered doctor she cannot be deregistered, and at the time of writing her paper has not been retracted. I should note here that, for many who read this, I will be seen as providing a defence for Andrew Wakefield and any defence would be seen as unforgivable. If you are a reader who has this response, I just ask that you step back a little from that response and look a little more closely at this controversy. I am not making any claim to support the idea that MMR causes autism. I have not undertaken any study of that. What is of interest here is the treatment of those who might raise even the possibility of such a connection.

Implementing vaccinations policies can too be a source of danger. Although vaccinations policies are broadly embraced in the Global North, in the Global South they may be a site of friction between opposing factions. This is most dramatically illustrated in the case of government employees in Pakistan tasked with administering polio vaccination programmes. Pakistan is one of the few countries in the world where polio is endemic. But in a four-year period from 2012, 71 administrators of the polio vaccination programme were killed by anti-government militants (Kakalia and Karrar 2016). In some countries, such as Pakistan and Nigeria, anti-vaccination sentiment can be vehement, with the procedure being portrayed as having any number of negative connotations, such as being anti-Islamic or being a covert form of birth control (Kakalia and Karrar 2016). The strategic use by the US Central Intelligence Agency of a fake vaccination campaign to obtain the DNA of the children of Osama Bin Laden in 2011 provided a rich resource for Pakistani militants to justify their attacks on polio vaccination programmes (The Lancet 2014).

## Concluding comments

Returning to Foucault's concept of biopolitics, we can consider the ways in which the technologies of vaccines and pharmaceuticals can integrate with other technologies to discipline and control populations. For example, vaccination certification is required in many countries for school entry purposes, and only medical exemptions may be allowed (Delamater *et al.* 2016). Registers of vaccine certification are subsequently created. Those who are recorded as being unvaccinated can be discriminated against and refused admittance to schools during epidemic outbreaks. The unvaccinated are seen as a risk as they may have disease, and so they need to be kept away to prevent contagion. In Foucault's language, the intervention of vaccines and the disciplining of populations that they are associated with are portrayed as a form of pastoral care, aimed at sustaining and improving the lives of everyone (Smart 1985), and so 'bio-power is spread under the banner of making people healthy and protecting them' (Dreyfus and Rabinow 1982: 195).

A particular feature of vaccinations is that they are bound up with extreme forms of governance, much more forceful than most other therapeutic approaches. Where the state determines that the population are not appropriately self-governing, further measures are taken to limit the choices that people can make and enforce vaccination schedules (Delamater *et al.* 2016). At the other extreme, vaccination programmes can become the target of those fighting the state, where force can be brutal and final (Kakalia and Karrar 2016).

The vaccination issue brings to the fore a number of governance processes that shines a light on the social organisation of state-sponsored therapeutic and preventive interventions. The endeavours to standardise populations so that everyone is treated in the same way allows for powerful forms of state control. Dissenters can be identified, isolated and vilified and at the same time the market for therapeutic products can be extensively expanded. There are then powerful forces at play to foster a form of governmentality based on a concern for longevity and health protection that can be applied to entire populations.

## References

Barrow, L. (2002). In the beginning was the lymph: The hollowing of stational vaccination in England and Wales, 1840–1898. In: *Medicine, Health and the Public Sphere in Britain, 1600–2000* (ed. S. Sturdy), 205–223. London and New York: Routledge.

Boseley, S. (2010). Andrew Wakefield struck off register by General Medical Council. *Guardian* (24 May).

Brunson, E. (2013). How parents make decisions about their children's vaccinations. *Vaccine* 13 (46): 5466–5470.

Chaitow, L. (1987). *Vaccination and Immunization: Dangers, Delusions and Alternatives.* Saffron Walden: C.W. Daniel.

Colgrove, J. (2002). The McKeown thesis: A historical controversy and its enduring influence. *American Journal of Public Health* 92 (5): 725–729.

Copp, N. and Zanella, A. (1992). *Discovery, Innovation and Risk: Case Studies in Science and Technology*. Cambridge, USA: MIT Press.

Cunha, M. and Durand, J.-Y. (2013). Anti-bodies: The production of dissent, *Ethnologia Europaea* 43 (1): 35–54.

Day, A. (2008). Child immunisation: Reactions and responses to New Zealand government policy 1920–1990. PhD dissertation. The University of Auckland.

Delamater, P., Leslie, T. and Yang, Y.T. (2016). A spatiotemporal analysis of non-medical exemptions from vaccination: California schools before and after SB277. *Social Science and Medicine* 168: 230–238.

DeLong, G. (2011). A positive association between autism prevalence and childhood vaccination uptake across the US population. *Journal of Toxicology and Environmental Health Part A* 74: 903–916.

Dew, K. (1999). Epidemics, panic and power: Representations of measles and measles vaccines. *Health* 3 (4): 379–398.

Dreyfus, H. and Rabinow, P. (1982). *Michel Foucault: Beyond Structuralism and Hermeneutics*. Brighton: Harvester Press.

Durbach, N. (2000). They might as well brand us: Working class resistance to compulsory vaccination in Victorian England. *Social History of Medicine* 13 (1): 45–62.

Durrheim, D. and Jones, A. (2016). Public health and the necessary limits of academic freedom? *Vaccine* 34 (22): 2467–2468.

Foucault, M. (1978). *The History of Sexuality: An Introduction*. Allen Lane: London.

Foucault, M. (1988). The political technology of individuals. In: *Technologies of the Self: A Seminar With Michel Foucault* (eds L. Martin, H. Gutman and P.H. Hutton). Amherst: University of Massachusetts Press.

Halliday, S. (2007). *The Great Filth: The War against Disease in Victorian England*. Chalford, Stroud: Sutton Publishing.

Hardy, A. (2001). *Health and Medicine in Britain Since 1860*. Houndmills: Palgrave.

Hobson-West, P. (2007). 'Trusting blindly can be the biggest risk of all': Organised resistance to childhood vaccination in the UK. *Sociology of Health and Illness*, 29 (2): 198–215.

Holton, A., Weberling, B., Clarke, C. and Smith, M. (2012). The blame frame: Media attribution of culpability about the MMR-autism vaccination scare. *Health Communication* 27 (7): 690–701.

Kakalia, S. and Karrar, H. (2016). Polio, public health, and the new pathologies of militancy in Pakistan. *Critical Public Health* 26 (4): 446–454.

Langmuir, A., Henderson, D., Serfling, R. and Sherman, I. (1962). The importance of measles as a health problem. *American Journal of Public Health and the Nations Health* 52 (suppl. 2), 1–4.

Leask, J. and Danchin, M. (2017). Imposing penalties for vaccine rejection requires strong scrutiny. *Journal of Paediatrics and Child Health*, 53 (5): 431–519.

Manca, T. (2018). 'One of the greatest medical success stories': Physicians and nurses' small stories about vaccine knowledge and anxieties. *Social Science and Medicine* 196: 182–189.

Martin, B. (1996). Sticking a needle into science: The case of polio vaccines and the origin of AIDS. *Social Studies of Science* 26 (2): 245–276.

Martin, B. (2013). When public debates become abusive. *Social Medicine* 7 (2): 90–97.

Martin, B. (2016). STS and researcher intervention strategies. *Engaging Science, Technology and Society* 2 (1): 55–66.

McKeown, T. (1979). *The Role of Medicine*. Oxford: Basil Blackwell.

Nelson, R. and Moser, J. (2008). Controversy surrounds Gardasil. *American Journal of Nursing* 108 (7): 17.

New, S.J. and Senior, M.L. (1991). 'I don't believe in needles': Qualitative aspects of a study into the uptake of infant immunisation in two English health authorities. *Social Science and Medicine* 33: 509–518.

Poltorak. M., Leach, M., Fairhead, J. and Cassell, J. (2005). 'MMR talk' and vaccination choices: An ethnographic study in Brighton. *Social Science and Medicine* 61 (3): 709–719.

Porter, T. (1995). *Trust in Numbers: The Pursuit of Objectivity in Science and Public Life.* Princeton: Princeton University Press.

Puliyel, J.M. and Madhavi, Y. (2008). Vaccines: Policy for public good or private profit. *Indian Journal of Medical Research* 127 (1): 1–3.

Scott, J.C. (1998). *Seeing Like a State: How Certain Schemes to Improve the Human Condition Have Failed.* New Haven and London: Yale University Press.

Smart, B. (1985). *Michel Foucault.* Chichester: Ellis Horwood.

Streefland, P. (2001). Public doubts about vaccination safety and resistance against vaccination. *Health Policy* 55: 159–172.

The Lancet (2014). Polio eradication. The CIA and their unintended victims. *The Lancet* 383 (9932): 1862.

Wigginton, B., Morphett, K. and Gartner, C. (2017). Differential access to health care and support? A qualitative analysis of how Australian smokers conceptualise and respond to stigma. *Critical Public Health* 27 (5): 577–590.

Wilyman, J. (2015). A critical analysis of the Australian government's rationale for its vaccination policy. PhD thesis. School of Humanities and Social Inquiry. University of Wollongong.

# 8 Adverse reactions and the proliferation of risk

The use of toxic materials for therapeutic effect has a very long tradition, and this is reflected in the Greek-derived term pharmakon, which can mean both poison and remedy (Riley 2010). The Hippocratic collection of works, associated with the famous Greek physician Hippocrates, noted up to 400 drugs used for therapeutic purposes, including the use of the toxic plants black hellebore as a purge and white hellebore as an emetic (Trease 1964). The development of systematic approaches to test the efficacy and safety of drugs did not occur until the twentieth century, but we should perhaps remain wary about the toxicity of the drugs we are prescribed and access. The consumption of drugs is an everyday occurrence for many people, with nearly half of all Americans taking at least one prescription drug in a given month; and 90 per cent of those over 65 taking at least one drug. The consumption of these toxic substances comes at a cost, with adverse reactions to medications accounting for 5 per cent of hospital admissions in the United States (US) (Hennessy and Strom 2015).

Antoine Lentacker (2016) suggests that pharmaceuticals act differently from other goods we purchase because they are goods 'for which the final judgment of experience is indefinitely deferred, and the dependence of users on discourse indefinitely prolonged' (Lentacker 2016: 142). This statement needs a bit of unpacking. What Lentacker suggests is that people cannot assess the qualities of drugs until they consume them. That is, it is only by taking the drug that you might be able to work out its effects on you. Does it work? Does it cause problems for you? But any uncertainties you have are not dispelled even with consumption, as the possibility of rare long-term adverse reactions are always there. Drug companies invest vast resources in developing positive discourses about their drugs. More money is spent on the marketing than on the development of drugs. Therefore signs, both visual and text-based, are crucially important in influencing consumers of drugs and potential users to deal with the uncertainties of drug consumption (Lentacker 2016).

The limited capacity of individuals to determine all the consequences of taking drugs might not be such a concern if we could trust the determinations of experts about the effectiveness and safety of drugs. But can we have such faith in the systems that have been developed around drug use? In this chapter, I suggest that, as drug development and marketing are driven by companies motivated by profit, our trust will at times be misplaced. Donald Light's diagnostic category of the risk proliferation syndrome captures why we should be concerned about the development and marketing of drugs (Light 2010).

## The risk proliferation syndrome

Developments in testing the safety and efficacy of pharmaceuticals would, on the surface, give comfort to those taking prescription or over-the-counter drugs, but since the thalidomide case, concerns over drug safety have been regularly raised. Why should this be the case if the regulatory agencies are ensuring that drugs are beneficial?

With a sense of mischievousness, Donald Light likens the development and marketing of pharmaceuticals to a disease, referring to it as risk proliferation syndrome. This concept suggests that there are increasing levels of risk that patients face in relation to pharmaceuticals, resulting from a number of factors. These factors include drug companies testing their own products, and regulatory reviewers having limited time to assess the data produced by drug companies. Pressure on the regulatory authorities, like the Food and Drug Administration (FDA), may mean a less than thorough assessment of applications is made. This, and the inevitable limitations of what clinical trials can tell us, means that drug companies can mass market products without knowing how safe or otherwise they are. The marketing of drugs and the propagation of disease models fostering the unnecessary consumption of drugs, noted in Chapter 3, further proliferates risk (Light 2010).

One pressure on those tasked with regulating drugs is that increasing safety and efficacy requirements in drug development has led to criticisms about the time lag in getting drugs to the market. The claim is that if there is a delay in getting a drug to the market people may die or have a lower quality of life. From this point of view, many deaths could be prevented if some drugs were fast tracked. In a study of all drugs approved by the FDA between 1993 and 2010, it was found that 17 drugs were approved and later withdrawn, and that those withdrawn drugs were prescribed at 112 million physician office visits (Saluja *et al.* 2016). That is, before the drugs were withdrawn they were very popular. The toxicities of the various withdrawn drugs included increased risk of heart attacks and strokes, fatal arrhythmia, hepatic failure and liver failure. Six of the withdrawn drugs had gained approval through the expedited review process. There are clearly risks to pharmaceutical users resulting from expedited reviews that need to be balanced against the gains promised from new drugs.

The fast tracking of drugs and the use of expedited reviews has led to more reliance on the post-marketing assessment of new drugs and reporting of adverse reactions to them (Weatherall 2006) – that is, to a greater reliance on pharmacovigilance mechanisms. Pharmacovigilance is the activity of 'analysing and managing the risk posed by medications once they have come on to the market' (Lopez-Gonzalez *et al.* 2009). We have to be vigilant in assessing the effects of pharmaceuticals. Fatal adverse drug reactions (ADRs) may be as high as the fourth leading cause of death in the US (Lazarou *et al.* 1998) constituting an important public health problem in terms of mortality, morbidity and cost (Lopez-Gonzalez *et al.* 2009). As a result of increasing concern to detect adverse drug events, many countries have developed pharmacovigilance systems to collect and monitor data on adverse reactions (Lopez-Gonzalez *et al.* 2009). The World Health Organization (WHO) Uppsala Monitoring Centre was set up in 1978 as yet another attempt to respond to the thalidomide tragedy (Uppsala Monitoring Centre 2018). It collects and assesses information from the pharma-covigilance systems of WHO member countries, and had received over 9 million case reports of suspected ADRs by 2014 (Uppsala Monitoriing Centre 2014). This is only a fraction of likely reportable ADRs, as 98 per cent of all reports come from high income countries. Given the high rate of ADRs pharmacovigi-lance activities are important.

One of the reasons that ADRs are only identified after drugs have come on to the market, aside from the issue of expedited review processes, is that even when the findings from randomised controlled trials (RCTs) suggest that the interven-tion is of benefit, known as efficacy, it is not known if these benefits will trans-late to the use of the drug when it is marketed, known as effectiveness. Efficacy requires that a clinical procedure achieve benefits to individuals in defined popu-lations when it is applied under ideal circumstances. Effectiveness applies to the clinical setting, not a controlled setting, where a procedure should do more good than harm. Many interventions found by RCT to be efficacious do not lead to improved outcomes when translated into practice (Glasgow *et al.* 1999). Patients on trials are specifically selected. They may not have the co-morbidities that patients prescribed the drug when it is on the market have, and may not use mul-tiple medications. The diversity of patients in the population does not match those of drug trials.

Light uses the example of Vioxx to illustrate a number of issues related to the risk proliferation syndrome (Light 2010). Vioxx was an anti-inflammatory pain-killer given US FDA approval in 1999 and marketed by Merck. It is estimated that in the US, Vioxx caused 88,000 to 130,000 heart attacks or strokes with up to 40 per cent mortality rate, making it, according to FDA officials, the greatest drug catastrophe in US history. The death toll worldwide is estimated to be more than double the US toll. The side effects of the drug, including heart attacks and strokes, were known three years before the drug was withdrawn, and Merck's own trials demonstrated cardiovascular risk from the drug. Not only did the drug company fail to convey its concern and bring the known risks to the attention of regulatory agencies, but it tried to censor doctors who were critical of the drug. Drug company sales representatives played down the risk of side effects in an aggressive marketing campaign in which millions of free samples were handed out to physicians. The FDA demanded that the company cease misrepresenting the drug in its advertising where benefits were overstated and risks understated. Merck responded by making some adjustments to their advertisements, but con-tinued its mass marketing campaign.

Although agencies like the FDA may try to exert some control over how medications are advertised by drug companies, they have no control over the pronouncements of academics and researchers in conferences and in articles. Scientific articles on the benefits of Vioxx, which were published in medical journals, were written by company-paid ghost writers. The use of ghost writers in promoting drugs is common practice. The development of ghost writers started to occur from the 1980s when drug companies began outsourcing medical writing to communication agencies (Healy 2006). By 1998, over 10 per cent of articles published in six established peer-reviewed journals were written by ghost writers (Healy 2006). Ghost writers can include company statisticians, commercial writers and others who do not appear as authors on the final article, thus hiding the input of drug company representatives (Goldacre 2012). Drug companies also pay expert members of the medical profession to act as opinion leaders. John Abraham documents how these opinion leaders may act as editors for special supplements of journals, with articles for these supplements receiving little independent peer review (Abraham 2009).

The Vioxx case demonstrates a number of features of the development and marketing of drugs that challenge the idea that we can rely on drugs that come on to the market. In the Vioxx case, the scientific activity of clinical trials could not be relied on, nor the representation of medical science in clinical journals. Even though the drug regulatory agencies made efforts to constrain Merck, they had limited success. John Abraham notes similar limitations in the capacity or regulatory agencies in the United Kingdom (UK). Premarketing safety testing and systems put in place to detect adverse reactions to drugs, such as the yellow card system, failed to prevent drug disasters in the 1970s and 1980s. The yellow card scheme was established in 1964 to allow health care professionals to spontaneously report ADRs to the Medicines and Healthcare products Regulatory Agency. Despite its existence, thousands of patients were adversely affected, including many deaths, from the beta-blocker Practolol and the anti-arthritis drug Opren (Abraham 2009). Abraham argues in relation to this and other cases that regulatory agencies reliance on yellow card data in the UK, or spontaneous reporting from health care professionals, produced low estimates of risk, highlighting that very few heart attacks as a result of the use of Vioxx were picked up by this system in the UK.

Drug regulatory agencies also have limited influence over experts who develop guidelines and make recommendations through such things as consensus conferences (Healy 2006). Guidelines and recommendations have been developed by panels of consultants with many of those experts having ties to the drug companies marketing the drugs that they are assessing (Healy 2006). David Healy, a psychiatrist, discusses the development of guidelines for antipsychotic medications that would lead to preferred drug listings on hospital formularies in the US. These guidelines influence consensus panels in other parts of the world, such as those undertaken by NICE (National Institute for Health and Care Excellence) in the UK. Guidelines that were developed supported the use of newer antipsychotic drugs that were no better than older drugs but approximately 80 times more expensive (Healy 2006). Guidelines developed by NICE for the use of these drugs not only lacked an evidence base but ignored the evidence that the newer antipsychotics produced significantly higher death and suicide rates (Healy 2006). Healy's interpretation of the development of guidelines suggests that we should be wary about them.

To counter the excessively rosy pictures of positive health outcomes from drugs, as promoted in drug company advertising, all advertising could be accompanied by appropriate warnings about side effects. In a well-publicised case, a lack of warning about side effects, including suicide, being associated with the psychotropic drug Paxil, led a jury to find GlaxoSmithKline, the drug manufacturer, guilty for failing to provide adequate information about side effects. The court case was taken after Donald Schell killed his wife, their daughter and granddaughter and then killed himself after going on the drug to treat depression. The jury awarded the family US$6.4 million in 2001 (Hilts 2001).

If we focus on such terrible outcomes from adverse reactions to drugs it would seem imperative to provide warnings to people when offered prescription medications. But there is another side to this argument. There is a great deal of stigma and fear associated with mental illness. People who may be helped by medications are already tentative about seeing health professionals and being given a label of having a mental illness. People can fear a whole range of things, such as a fear of losing control over their own decisions and lives, a fear of the medications, fear of having to confront oneself and a fear of being judged (Dew *et al.* 2007). Adding a warning that the medications may be bad for you may be yet another incentive to avoid seeking help (Williams and Donaghue 2010). This tension between disclosing information about risks and encouraging people to take potentially beneficial drugs applies to many pharmaceuticals, and we will see examples of this in clinical consultation rooms in the following chapter. The pharmakon nature of drugs, being both a poison and a remedy, is entwined with drug companies pursuing profits, exacerbating the dilemmatic nature of drug consumption.

The risks associated with drug development and marketing do not fall evenly across populations. For a whole host of reasons, there will be different health outcomes and adverse reactions to drugs related to age, class, gender, ethnicity, sexuality and so on. The risks associated with contraceptive drugs is a very clear-cut example bringing into focus the gendered nature of risk assessment and information by drug regulation agencies, the drug industry and others. Alina Geampana provides an insightful illustration of this in her analysis of how state drug regulating agencies and medical associations responded to a controversy over an oral contraceptive drug called Drospirenone marketed variously as Yaz and Yasmin (Geampana 2016). The drug became a focus of controversy with media reporting of deaths from blood clots following the use of the drug. The drug was linked to 23 deaths in Canada and over 100 in the US.

Geampana notes that there has been a long history of epidemiological studies identifying links between oral contraceptives and blood clots, as well as other serious health conditions. Drug agency reviews of Drospirenone found that it was associated with a 1.5–3 times higher risk of blood clots than other contraceptive pills. The FDA and medical associations used a number of strategies to downplay this concern. One was identifying potential methodological flaws in the epidemiological studies that came up with negative findings. Another was to emphasise that, even with its higher risk profile, taking the drug was less likely to cause blood clots than pregnancy. This sets up a very simple dichotomy for women: with their risky bodies, taking a drug is less risky than getting pregnant. Geampana notes that comparisons between Drospirenone and other less risky oral contraceptives was downplayed, and that all the other potential side effects from oral contraceptives (such as migraines, weight gain, loss of libido) were not mentioned at all by these agencies when responding to the controversy. In sum, we can suggest that, as women's bodies are constructed as being naturally and inevitably sites or risk, therefore more risks can be taken with those bodies as compared to the male body.

To summarise here, the risk of negative health impacts from drugs is amplified by a number of processes captured by Light in his concept of the risk proliferation syndrome. Drugs come to the market with limited knowledge about their effectiveness; they are promoted in ways that defy control by drug regulating agencies; and some groups in society will be more exposed to the risks posed by drugs than others. The hazards presented by drug consumption have their gestation well before they come on to the market, and it is to the premarketing phase of drug trajectories, the clinical trial, to which I will now turn.

## Clinical trials

Clinical trials of pharmaceuticals can promote the proliferation of risk on a number of grounds. They pose a direct danger to those who participate in the trial. Trial participants can be selected in such a way as to give a false sense of the safety or efficacy of a drug. In addition, pharmaceutical companies can use a number of strategies to present an overly positive picture of trial outcomes.

Clinical trials do not only pose a risk for those who base drug consumption decisions on trial findings. In the first instance, they pose a risk for those who participate in the trials. Risks for trial participants are arguably justifiable if the likelihood of determining clinical benefit is high, but this is perhaps rarely the case as most drugs that are tested are likely to have only marginal benefit if they get to the market (Yusuf *et al.* 2008). In some cases there have been suggestions of moral irresponsibility on the part of drug companies. For example, in January 2016 a phase 1 trial of a drug, BIA-10–2474, was conducted in France. A phase 1 trial is when a drug is tested for the first time in healthy humans. BIA-10–2474 had no clear potential to provide therapeutic value, and the trial led to the death of one healthy volunteer and serious neurological damage for three others. The trial used ascending doses of the drug, but the increases were steep and high doses were given. Nicholas Moore (2016) suggests that one possible reason for the high dose is that the drug company was on a fishing expedition to try to find some kind of activity that might have therapeutic value. But this came at a high cost for volunteers. Another widely publicised example of harm caused to volunteers in trials occurred in Northwick Park Hospital in 2006 when six men suffered multiple organ failure (Brown and Calnan 2010).

Undertaking clinical trials is an expensive exercise, even if drug companies exaggerate the expense. When RCTs were first used to test drug efficacy and safety, they were funded by governments and conducted by academics. Today, government-funded trials are very much in the minority; the majority of trials are funded and conducted by the pharmaceutical industry (Yusuf *et al.* 2008). There are a number of reasons why trials are expensive. One is that the new drugs are likely to have only moderate benefits over other drugs or over placebo, if they have any benefit at all. In order to detect small benefits, very large trials need to be conducted, which might involve many thousands of subjects escalating the costs of trials for these new drugs (Yusuf *et al.* 2008). Other costs include approval processes prior to the trials being conducted, costs associated with recruiting subjects, costs of running the trial, costs of meeting quality assurance specifications and so on. In order to reduce the cost of clinical trials, drug companies may use private research groups or for-profit organisations instead of traditional academic research groups.

Although drug trials may be randomised, the selection of who is included in the study can have a major role in determining what is found. Adriana Petryna's (Petryna 2007) extensive research on clinical trials uncovered claims by scientific officers of contract research organisations, who oversee the conduct of clinical trials that, companies would select specific populations in order to improve the chances of identifying drug benefits and avoiding the identification of side effects. This is exacerbated by the increasing tendency to conduct RCTs for pharmaceuticals in what are termed 'non-traditional' research areas (for example, Latin America and Eastern Europe) by commercial companies (Petryna 2007). Petryna (2007: 24) reports a scientific advisor of a contract research organisation stating that 'companies can now pick and choose populations in order to get a most pronounced drug benefit signal as well as a "no-harm" signal'. This is achieved through trial recruitment strategies, which, for example, can recruit from treatment-naive groups with very little history of pharmaceutical use, whilst the results are generalised to apply to treatment-saturated markets where many people are on multiple medications (Petryna 2007). Given the likelihood of interactions between pharmaceuticals the treatment-saturated populations may react very differently to the trial drug than those who participated in the trial, and so adverse reactions may not be detected until the drugs are marketed.

Martin (2006) suggests that the extensive list of potential side effects found on the thin, fragile paper inserts inside the drug packet, are most likely generated from these trials that have been undertaken on people in poorer countries with less access to compensation systems. She suggests that we, collectively, are able to displace this issue that the drugs for our benefit 'contain the blood of others spilt in clinical trials' (Martin 2006: 286). Not only do trials provide limited information on the benefits of drugs, the information comes at a cost to the people who are effectively out of sight and out of mind.

Drug companies use other strategies to manipulate trials. Often trials are between a new drug and a drug of choice that is already on the market. New antipsychotic drugs that came onto the market in the 1990s were compared to an older antipsychotic drug, haloperidol, in premarketing trials. All the trials used a comparator dose of haloperidol that was higher than necessary for it to be efficacious and therefore produced more side effects. This tactic promoted the chance that their drugs would have a better side effect profile than haloperidol (Healy 2006). Another strategy is to use cut-off points for reporting that can hide high levels of side effects. In trials of the antidepressant sertraline, used for the treatment of depressed children, a trial found a 9 per cent rate of suicidality in the depressed children when taking the drug. However, this was not reported. The article on this trial only reported side effects that were at a rate of 10 per cent or higher (Healy 2006). Another strategy reported by Healy (2006) is to use pre-screening of participants, with clinical trials of fluoxetine screening out more than 80 per cent of the patients from entering the study (Healy 2006). In trials on Prozac, participants who reacted adversely to the drug were dropped from the trial in a test phase, excluding their data from the results (Healy 2006). These are some of the ways in which trials can be used to provide an overly positive picture of drug safety and efficacy.

Petryna argues that companies conducting clinical trials of medications operate within a 'paradigm of expected failure' (Petryna 2007: 33). That is, there is limited focus on the prevention of problems with medications before they go to market, particularly in identifying any long-term issues as trials tend to be short-term. As such, failure in terms of the safety of medications is expected by the drug companies. Even in what might appear to be a strong drug regulatory environment problems with drugs won't be identified until after they come on to the market.

## Selective publication

Once trials have been completed we might expect that the results would be published, either in a medical journal or some other forum. This is not always the case. There are many reasons for this, including the withholding of trial data by either the drug companies or other scientists, the dependence of medical journals on drug company advertising and support, and the limited efficacy of drug trial registers.

The withholding of trial data can take many forms, with a range of motivations. Drug companies have been known to avoid declaring the side effects of drugs identified during clinical trials, as has been noted with the Vioxx case. Drug companies have been able to influence perceptions through the selective publication of data. For example, published data on the clinical trials of the antidepressant Reboxetine (Edronaz) showed that it was better than placebo and as good as other antidepressants, and was approved for use by the UK's Medicines and Healthcare products Regulatory Agency. The positive effect demonstrated and published in medical journals was based on only one trial out of the seven that were undertaken. The unpublished data from the other six trials showed it was less effective, with greater risk of side effects (Goldacre 2012).

In 2011, the *British Medical Journal* published research on reporting bias in clinical trials. Of the 59 clinical trial investigators who participated in the study, 16 admitted failure to report clinical trial outcomes that had been analysed, and 17 collected data that was not subsequently analysed. In many cases, the failure to report outcomes was based on a view that the findings were uninteresting or were negative, or that the reader would miss the important message if all the data were reported. The following quote from a trial investigator is informative:

> When we looked at the data, it actually showed an increase in harm amongst those who got the active treatment, and we ditched it because we weren't expecting it … there doesn't appear to be a kind of framework or a mechanism for understanding this association and therefore you know people didn't have faith that this was a valid finding … so we buried it.
>
> (Smyth *et al.* 2011)

This quote suggests that the selective publication of data is not always motivated by drug companies determined to get their products on to the market. Selective publication can be motivated by scientists working within a particular paradigm. It is noted in Chapter 1 that when scientists work within a particular paradigm or thought collective, then any exceptions to what is expected within that paradigm need to be explained away. This is required so that the particular way of thinking that the scientists have been socialised into, which is the basis of their understanding of how the world works, is not challenged or undermined. In this example, we see scientists discarding any findings that do not conform to their paradigm.

Medical journals have been criticised for not successfully keeping an arms distance from pharmaceutical companies. One reason for this is that medical journals are dependent upon drug company advertising. Additionally, drug companies can generate revenue for medical journals by purchasing reprints of articles that are supportive of their products. For example, Merck paid the *New England Journal of Medicine* US$900,000 for reprints of one article on a Vioxx trial (Brody 2010).

In response to concerns about the conduct of clinical trials, attempts have been made to establish clinical trial registers. Protocols of clinical trials are made available through these registers, to allow checking of whether those protocols were adhered to and if the trial data was published. Registers have been established in the US and Europe, and a number of prestigious medical journals have published policies stating that they would not publish clinical trials unless the trials had been properly registered. In the US in 2007, the FDA passed an amendment requiring registration of all trials and the posting of trial results for any drug marketed after 2007. Although this should ease disquiet over selective publication, research has shown that medical journals have not adhered to their policy statements, with only half of the published trials having been adequately registered, and only one-fifth of the trials in the US required to register results have actually done so (Goldacre 2012).

Selective publication means that it is not possible for drug regulatory agencies, health professionals, or users of pharmaceuticals to gather together all relevant information that might be relevant to decision-making about drug use.

## Undermining research

In addition to manipulating the collection and publication of data, pharmaceutical companies have a history of actively undermining or repressing research that challenges their interests. In the late 1970s, Boehringer Ingelheim marketed Fenoterol, a high dose beta agonist preparation used as an asthma medication. Marketing was particularly successful in New Zealand, but epidemiologists noted a correspondence between the increase in the market share of Fenoterol and an increase in asthma deaths. They proposed a Fenoterol hypothesis: that the medication was the cause for the increase in mortality (Pearce 1992). Research was undertaken, and the results suggested that Fenoterol use caused cardiac side effects. A paper was prepared for *The Lancet*, and after independent review it was accepted for publication. Subsequent lobbying from the drug company led the journal to withdraw the unconditional publication of the paper, but after further representations from the researchers, *The Lancet* relented, again agreeing to accept the paper for publication. Upon publication, Boehringer Ingelheim sent out packages to doctors, pharmacists, health reporters and others undermining the findings of the research and so encouraging the continued use of Fenoterol. Further studies confirmed the original research findings, and Fenoterol was eventually removed from the drug tariff, leading to a decline in asthma deaths.

In another case of undermining research, in 1999 GlaxoSmithKline (GSK) gained FDA approval for Rosiglitazone, marketed as Avandia, as a treatment for type 2 diabetes. It became the bestselling anti-diabetes drug in the world. Pre-approval studies had shown an excess of cardiovascular events from use of the drug, and GSK had conducted its own study that showed that a competitor's drug was safer, but this data was kept secret. Researchers were able to obtain data from GSK, and through their analysis demonstrated that the drug caused up to a 43 per cent increase in the risk of heart problems. The researchers submitted an article based on the findings to the *New England Journal of Medicine*. A copy of the submitted manuscript was immediately circulated to the company who, although finding no basis to disagree with the findings, organised a public relations process to undermine the findings. Later work confirmed the concerns about the drug, and it was removed from the market or restricted in use in 2010 (Goldacre 2012; Nissen 2013).

A well-publicised case of suppression involved a researcher who reported adverse effects from Deferiprone, a drug developed by Apotex for the treatment of a blood disorder. The company had co-funded the research into Deferiprone, but threatened the researcher, Nancy Olivieri, with legal action if she disclosed her concerns about the drug. Olivieri did report her findings to scientific meetings and had them published in academic journals. Due to pressure from the company, she was removed as director of the research programme at the University of Toronto (Nathan and Weatherall 1999). In response to international pressure however, the University restored Olivieri to a teaching and research position (Savage 2000).

Attempts by drug companies to suppress the work of researchers who uncover findings that threaten the market of the companies' drugs are yet another element that proliferates drug risks.

## Concluding comments

In this chapter I have presented material that might challenge our faith in regulatory agencies and in trials testing the efficacy and safety of pharmaceuticals. At the heart of this issue is the way in which the science of pharmaceutical testing is shaped and conducted. Attempts have been made by social theorists to demarcate the practices of ethical science from unethical science. One well-cited endeavour at demarcation was undertaken by sociologist Robert Merton, who was particularly concerned to show Nazi science as a perversion of science. He wanted to claim that for a science to live up to its label, it must be free of political, ideological and economic interests in order to pursue its task of discovering the truth about the natural world.

He posited four norms of science: communism, universalism, disinterestedness and organised scepticism. The norm of communism stipulates that scientists share their findings: there must be a free exchange of ideas, and intellectual property is limited to peer recognition of one's contributions. Diffusion of results is encouraged by the recognition conferred, and this recognition is contingent upon publication. Universalism is a norm stipulating that merit is based on universal and impersonal criteria, and not criteria such as race, gender and class. Disinterestedness stipulates that one's self-interested behaviour is not to conflict with the goal of science. Finally, organised scepticism stipulates that the scientist should suspend judgement until sufficient evidence is available, but subject ideas to close scrutiny. Scientists are supposed to behave in this way because of their deep devotion to the advancement of knowledge (Merton 1973). The science of drug testing clearly breaches many of these norms, particularly those of communism, disinterestedness and organised scepticism. The science of drug testing would very often be, on Merton's assessment, a perversion of science. This perverted science shapes personal and policy decisions about pharmaceutical use.

The material covered in this chapter is an obvious challenge to market solutions to drug regulation. A market solution, that is, letting drug companies regulate themselves in response to consumer demand, not state regulation, might be appropriate in a situation where information was freely exchanged and widely accessible. What we have seen however are strategies deployed to conceal negative findings from drug trials. Sociologist Jürgen Habermas suggested that communication is an important feature in promoting a truly democratic society. The goal of undistorted communication, where knowledge or decisions are based on the force of the better argument, can occur in what he called the ideal speech situation. In an ideal type situation power and ideology does not distort communicative interaction between people. This potential for non-coerced debate amongst equals was the normative standard that Habermas sought to promote (Baert 2005). If non-coerced and non-distorted communication of research findings in relation to drugs could be achieved, then calls for de-regulating the pharmaceutical industry might have some basis. But the ideal speech situation does not exist when the profit motive and the role of financial capital (which will be discussed further in Chapter 11) so powerfully distort the information that people have access to. Our decisions about therapeutic choices and pharmaceutical practices are built on the distortions in communication confounded by the profit motivation of drug companies.

The consultation between pharmaceutical prescribers and users is one place where we might expect to see discussion of side effects, without the direct and immediate influence of drug companies. Health professionals are not usually drug company employees, and have been trained to critically reflect on diagnoses and prescriptions. Usually they will not make money from prescriptions and so the profit motive for prescribing a drug and for downplaying any adverse effects of drugs is absent. There are, however, other social forces that limit the recognition and acknowledgement of adverse reactions from pharmaceuticals in the consultation, and these forces are the focus on the next chapter.

# References

Abraham, J. (2009). Partial progress: Governing the pharmaceutical industry and the NHS, 1948–2008. *Journal of Health Politics Policy and Law* 34 (6): 931–977.

Baert, P. (2005). *Philosophy of the Social Sciences: Towards Pragmatism.* Cambridge: Polity Press.

Brody, H. (2010). The commercialization of medical decisions: Physicians and patients at risk. In: *The Risks of Prescription Drugs* (ed. D. Light), 70–90. New York: Columbia University Press.

Brown, P. and Calnan, M. (2010). Braving a faceless new world? Conceptualizing trust in the pharmaceutical industry and its products. *Health* 16 (1): 57–75.

Dew, K., Morgan, S., Dowell, A., McLeod, D., Bushnell, J. and Collings, S. (2007). 'It puts things out of your control': Fear of consequences as a barrier to patient disclosure of mental health issues to general practitioners. *Sociology of Health and Illness* 29 (7): 1059–1074.

Geampana, A. (2016). Pregnancy is more dangerous than the pill: A critical analysis of professional responses to the Yaz/Yasmin controversy. *Social Science and Medicine* 166: 9–16.

Glasgow, R., Vogt, T. and Boles, S. (1999). Evaluating the public health impact of health promotion interventions: The RE-AIM framework. *American Journal of Public Health* 89: 1322–1327.

Goldacre, B. (2012). *Bad Pharma: How Medicine is Broken and How We Can Fix It.* London: Fourth Estate.

Healy, D. (2006). Manufacturing consensus. *Culture, Medicine and Psychiatry* 30: 135–156.

Hennessy, S. and Strom, B. (2015). Improving postapproval drug safety surveillance: Getting better information sooner. *Annual Review of Pharmacology and Toxicology* 55: 75–87.

Hilts, P. (2001). Jury awards $6.4 million in killings tied to drug. *New York Times.* www.nytimes.com/2001/06/08/us/jury-awards-6.4-million-in-killings-tied-to-drug.html (accessed 29 November 2017).

Lazarou, J., Pomeranz, B.H. and Corey, P.N. (1998). Incidence of adverse drug reactions in hospitalized patients: A meta-analysis of prospective studies. *Journal of the American Medical Association* 279 (15): 1200–1205.

Lentacker, A. (2016). The symbolic economy of drugs. *Social Studies of Science* 46 (1): 140–156.

Light, D. (2010). Bearing the risks of prescription drugs. In: *The Risks of Prescription Drugs* (ed. D. Light), 1–39. New York: Columbia University Press.

Lopez-Gonzalez, E., Herdeiro, M.T. and Figueiras, A. (2009). Determinants of under-reporting of adverse drug reactions: A systematic review. *Drug Safety* 32 (1): 19–31.

Martin, E. (2006). The pharmaceutical person. *BioSocieties* 1 (3): 273–287.

Merton, R.K. (1973). *The Sociology of Science: Theoretical and Empirical Investigations.* Chicago and London: The University of Chicago Press.

Moore, N. (2016). Lessons from the fatal French study BIA-10-2474: Do not test in humans drugs that lack an identified therapeutic potential. *British Medical Journal* 353: i2727.

Nathan, D. and Weatherall, D. (1999). Academia and industry: Lessons from the unfortunate events in Toronto. *The Lancet* 353 (9155): 771.

Nissen, S. (2013). Rosiglitazone: A case of regulatory hubris. *British Medical Journal* 347.

Pearce, N. (1992). Adverse reactions: The fenoterol saga. In: *In For Health or Profit? Medicine, the Pharmaceutical Industry, and the State in New Zealand* (ed. P. Davis), 75–97. Auckland: Oxford University Press.

Petryna, A. (2007). Clinical trials offshored: On private sector science and public health. *BioSocieties* 2: 21–40.

Riley, A.T. (2010). *Godless Intellectuals? The Intellectual Pursuit of the Sacred Reinvented.* New York and Oxford: Berghahn.

Saluja, S., Woolhandler, S., Himmelstein, D., Bor, D. and McCormick, D. (2016). Unsafe drugs were prescribed more than one hundred million times in the United States before being recalled. *International Journal of Health Services* 44 (3): 523–530.

Savage, D. (2000). Academic freedom and institutional autonomy in New Zealand universities. In: *In Troubled Times: Academic Freedom in New Zealand* (ed. R. Crozier), 13–225. Palmerston North: Dunmore Press.

Smyth, R.M.D., Kirkham, J.J., Jacoby, A., Altman, D.G., Gamble, C. and Williamson, P.R. (2011). Frequency and reasons for outcome reporting bias in clinical trials: Interviews with trialists. *British Medical Journal* 342. 10.1136/bmj.c7153.

Trease, G. (1964). *Pharmacy in History.* London: Balliére, Tindall and Cox.

Uppsala Monitoriing Centre. (2014). *Uppsala Reports 66.* Uppsala: Uppsala Monitoring Centre.

Uppsala Monitoring Centre. (2018). Our story. www.who-umc.org/about-us/our-story/ (accessed 18 January 2018).

Weatherall, M. (2006). Drug treatment and the rise of pharmacology. In: *The Cambridge History of Medicine* (ed. R. Porter), 211–237. Cambridge: Cambridge University Press.

Williams, A. and Donaghue, N. (2010). 'Now that's a fair dinkum academic debate, but this affects people's lives': A discursive analysis of arguments for and against the provision of warnings about potential side effects of SSRIs in a public debate. *Critical Public Health* 20 (1): 15–24.

Yusuf, S., Bosch, J., Devereaux, P., Collins, R., Baigent, C., Granger, C., Califf, R. and Temple, R. (2008). Sensible guidelines for the conduct of large randomized trials. *Clinical Trials* 5 (1): 38–39.

# 9 Underreporting of side effects

## The underreporting of side effects

This chapter looks at how concerns about the side effects of prescribed pharmaceuticals are considered in the consultation. If you are a regular user of pharmaceutical medications there is a good chance that you would have had some sort of side effect to the medication, as this is a common experience. Side effects are a major health concern, but they are substantially underreported to pharmacovigilance agencies. Pharmacovigilance is the managing of the risks of pharmaceuticals once they are on the market. I argue that what can be observed in the consultation helps to explain why side effects are underreported to pharmacovigilance centres. If we, as a society, are concerned about improving pharmacovigilance, then the general practice consultation may not be the best place to focus our attention, and the following chapter further develops this argument.

I first became interested in looking at side effects when I was undertaking some research with colleagues looking at interactions between health professionals and patients. In this research, our team obtained video and audio recordings of consultations, and we were particularly interested in using the methodology of conversation analysis to explore these consultations. The initial research issues we were wanting to explore in relation to the data were how protocols to determine if a patient could access elective surgery were used, and what happened as a patient went from primary care (seeing their general practitioner – GP) to seeing a specialist and possibly on to surgery (see Dew *et al.* 2010: for some of the results of this research). To explore these topics we collected many consultations, and a whole range of other issues started coming to our attention. During the research we were asked by PHARMAC, an agency that manages the list of pharmaceuticals that are subsidised by the state in New Zealand, if we would be interested in presenting at their workshops. Our research team decided to take up this offer, and looked at our data for material that would be of interest to the PHARMAC audience. I decided to look at how side effects were talked about in the consultation.

Once I started to pull the cases together it became clear to me that there was something very interesting going on here. Using conversation analysis facilitated an interpretation indicating that GPs often presented side effects concerns about a drug they were prescribing in a rather vague way, and that patients were even vaguer when they raised concerns about side effects from prescribed medications. Patients' vaguely presented concerns tended to be downgraded by the GP. This suggested to our research team that it was interactionally difficult to have side effects recognised in the consultations. We then looked at the literature on side effects, and found that there was evidence of a massive underreporting of side effects. For example, it is estimated that up to 94 per cent of adverse drug reactions (ADRs) go unreported (Hazell and Shakir 2006). In the United States (US), it has been estimated that in 2005 there were 46 million ADRs experienced, but only 1 per cent of these were reported to the Food and Drug Administration (FDA) (Light 2010). Even serious adverse reactions are underreported with only 10 per cent of them spontaneously reported (Spelsberg *et al.* 2017). We thought we had found a piece of the puzzle that would help explain the underreporting, which related to the specific interactional requirements in the consultation. I will take you through our research on this shortly, but before doing that it is worth dwelling for a moment on the reception we had to our interpretation.

After the workshop we worked up a paper for potential publication and sent it off to a well-known journal of general practice. The paper was sent out for review and reviewers raised a few issues that would have been easy to respond to. However, the editor of the journal did not give us that opportunity, and rejected the paper. The reason he gave for rejecting the paper was that what we had observed was not something that happened in his own practice, the assumption being that either we were not really telling the truth or we had obtained some sort of particularly unusual sample. This was quite a surprise to me. The use of conversation analysis allows us to slow down the action that takes place in consultation, and so start to identify aspects of interactions that participants are not likely to be aware of. Our GP participants were not aware of what was happening (we had one GP on our research team – Anthony Dowell), and it is very unlikely that the editor of the journal would be aware of what was happening in his own consultations. This kind of reception from GPs to our interpretation occurred on other occasions. At an international conference in Switzerland an American family physician came up to me after our presentation and said what we presented was all very interesting, but it was not what happened in his practice. Similarly, at a local presentation, a GP who had an interest in, and experience of, using conversation analysis said to me that our interpretation was wrong. We discussed this at some length, and he soon apologised to me as he came to see his response as a 'knee jerk' reaction.

These anecdotes on the reception of our research are instructive. It suggests that GPs downgrading patient concerns about side effects is professionally unacceptable. Health professionals wanted to explain away the findings or claim that the findings were not relevant to them. This suggests that it is not easy for those who oversee the bulk of pharmaceutical prescribing in many countries, and who have a responsibility to identify and report side effects, to reflect on the impact of their own actions in this regard.

So now to some of the research. In our data set at the time we had 105 consultations. Side effects were talked about in 54 of those consultations, and there were 88 sequences of talk. There were 31 instances where patients associated adverse symptoms with a prescribed medication. Our starting point was to look at how this reporting was done. From our analysis of the data we considered two very prominent socio-medical dilemmas that shaped the outcomes of the interaction. One is that GPs act to persuade patients to accept and take prescribed medications whilst making them aware of possible side effects. The second is that patients who raise concerns about side effects work to avoid challenging the expertise of the GP and blaming the GP for what he or she has prescribed. These combine to act as a powerful mechanism for downgrading concerns about side effects and limiting their reporting to pharmacovigilance agencies. The interactional demand of the consultation is then one mechanism that promotes the underreporting of side effects.

## Patient associations of side effects and symptoms

In our data, we found that in the majority of cases where patients raised the possibility that a symptom they were experiencing related to a prescribed medication, the GP either provided no response to the patient or provided a negative response. An example of a negative response is where a patient reports recent weight gain and says 'I was just wondering if it was the medication', and the GP responds by saying 'no it shouldn't'. (For those not familiar with analysing conversations, there is a tendency for natural conversation not to follow formal language conventions).

By looking closely at how patients presented their concerns, it was clear that it was common for them to present them in a very indirect way, with what can be termed indirect discourse strategies (for a fuller discussion of this research see Dew *et al.* 2012). The following extract illustrates this.

The patient in this example has presented with a chronic rash. He has sought advice for this condition on previous occasions, receiving conflicting advice from other doctors and treatment, which has proved ineffective. After recounting this history, he implies that the rash may have been a reaction to a course of terbinafine (Lamisil) prescribed by this GP about a year ago. (The appendix at the end of this chapter provides some information on the conversation analysis transcription conventions used here).

---

**Textbox 9.1 Rash side effects transcript**

`GP02-08`

```
1 PT: I've got a rash (.) which um (2) is getting worse
2 GP: ok yep
3     ((lines omitted))
4 PT: it's in its (.) big phase at the moment it's active phase
5     but) its spreading round inside my leg so (.) it's time to
6     (.) do something about that
```

```
 7 GP: it's been there over a year hasn't it
 8 PT: yep
 9 GP: yep
10 PT: it- it actually started after um (.) I think you (.) I
11     came- the first time I saw you I had that problem with the
12     um (.) rash on my toes and stuff and you gave me a
13     prescription for er (2) the er foot stuff (.) couple of
14     big horse pills
15 GP: yep lamisil
16 PT: lamisil that's [right  ] so (.) I finished that=
17 GP:               [yep yep]
18 PT: =and it started up round about the same sort of time
19 GP: was june oh three that's interesting (.) if it was a (.)
20     reaction to the (.) tablets which I mean you can get a
21     reaction to any of them it- it- you wouldn't expect it to
22     carry on [(      ) um]
23 PT:         [no so it's] it seems to be a permanent feature
24     now
```

The circumspect and cautious presentation of the patient's concern is seen clearly here. The patient does not make an explicit claim that the medication (Lamisil) is the cause of the problem. Rather, he states that the GP gave him a prescription and the problem 'started up around about the same sort of time' (Line 18). Virginia Gill and Douglas Maynard refer to this type of presentation as a non-attributive tacit linkage proposal (Gill and Maynard 2006). These tacit explanations do not have a 'because' statement (e.g. 'I have got the rash because of Lamisil'); rather they use 'and' or 'but' constructions. Through this tactic, the patient avoids overtly proposing that the prescribed medication caused the rash. The conclusion is suggested but not explicitly stated. This is a common strategy when patients are offering their own problem explanations in the face of the expertise of the practitioner (Gill and Maynard 2006).

We can also see that the patient is doing some repair work before the proposal. A repair is a conversational mechanism that is used to deal with some trouble or difficulty. There may be a problem in hearing what is said, or in speaking and getting the right words, or in understanding (Schegloff *et al.* 1977). On Lines 10 and 11 the patient provides a self-initiated repair, stating 'it – it actually started after um (.) I think you (.) I came – the first time I saw you I had that problem'. The repair to find the 'best' way of speaking suggests that there is some trouble or problem that the patient is dealing with. He first seems to be going to say something like 'it actually started after you gave me that pill'. This would be a stronger version of the tacit linkage proposal, but for the patient this seems to be too strong, so he starts to move to what might be something like 'I think you gave me that pill'. Again this seems to be too strong, perhaps because of its accusatory nature with 'you gave', or the assumption that the patient is allowed to think about causation in consultations where doctors have the right to diagnose. So the patient stops and tries again to move away from presenting the GP as doing something active, like prescribing, to the patient doing something active, like coming in with a problem. Patients can appropriately and defensibly do that, go to a doctor with a problem. This all happens very quickly, and the patient appears to be working quite hard to find the right way to make the proposal.

The patient and the GP both invoke a time dimension to sanction their conclusions. For the patient, the problem 'started up around the same sort of time'. The patient's hedges of 'around about' and 'sort of' can, on one reading, be seen as vague and imprecise. Alternatively, they can also be read as doing a particular form of interactional work – functioning as a face-saving device for both participants (Goffman 1967). To save face is to protect the dignity or social value of yourself or of the person or people you are interacting with (Goffman 1967; Manning 1992). The patient is providing the GP with options to contest the timing, and at the same time providing himself with an escape if his implicit claim is rejected by the GP.

The clinician immediately recognises what is being proposed here and moves to provide reasons for rejecting the proposal. The rejection is done with a delicacy so that the proposal is not positioned as unreasonable, for example, seen in Lines 20 and 21 where the GP says 'you can get a reaction to any of them'. However, at the same time he implies that the causal relationship is unlikely. The statement that reactions *can* occur saves face for the patient before the GP delivers his rationale for minimising any association – 'you wouldn't expect it to carry on' (Lines 21–22). At this point the patient affiliates with the GP by stating that it is now a 'permanent feature' (Line 23), and does not offer any challenge to the GP's interpretation. Neither the patient nor the doctor pursues the side effects explanation for the rash from this point.

In our research, we did not make any claims about the likelihood of patient concerns being feasible. We were more interested in the process of presentation and how it was responded to. However, a common side effect of the drug the patient was concerned about is a rash. When the GP did come back to the issue of the rash later in the consultation, he did not suggest that it could be caused by the drug, he suggested that it was 'exacerbated' by stress. According to this explanation, stress is exacerbating something that was already present, the rash, but an explanation for the initial cause of the rash is not provided.

This next extract provides a contrasting example where a GP positively acknowledges the patient's association between a complaint and a medication, despite in the first instance proffering a contrasting proposal. The patient presents with a symptom that could, from a clinical perspective, be explained by a number of causes, with side effects to the drug coming towards the bottom of the list.

---

**Textbox 9.2 Vertigo transcript**

GP04-02

```
1 PT: I just- woke up and my head was just going round and round
2     and round … I just had (.) an incredible vertigo (.) that
3     made me feel quite ill (.) um (.) and then it sort of went
4     away although I am still a little bit (.) you know I don't
```

```
 5         sort of rush to (.) throw my head around
 6 GP: mm hm
 7 PT: um (.) I wondered if it was something to do with that m-
 8         ah anti malaria drug that (.) that the specialist has put
 9         me on
10         ((lines omitted))
11 GP: and do you feel nauseous with [it  ] yeah
12 PT:                                [yeah]
13         ((This is followed by further detail on the symptoms and
14         the GP pronounces that the condition is vertigo))
15 GP: well there are a number of different causes one of the
         commonest is a virus
16 PT: all right
17 GP: mm
18 PT: so it could of been the start of this virus
19 GP: yeah though that would (.) yeah that's possible but it (.)
20         you know it's not sort of typical for what's going round
21         at the moment
22 PT: oh okay
23 GP: so when y- when you (.) (but) we'll come- maybe come back
24         to that (.) when the cold started what did it- what
25         symptoms did you start off with
```

The patient presents her suggestion of a link between the drug and her symptoms in a tentative way: 'I wondered if it was something to do with that m- ah anti malaria drug' (Lines 7–9). She provides an implicit contrast proposal, stating, 'I should get my ears checked and things like that' (not shown) – thus, providing another possible explanation for her symptoms. In this case the drug was not prescribed by the GP but by a specialist, so any threat is not to the GP personally. After a further elaboration on the symptoms by the patient (Lines omitted) the GP inquires about the symptoms: 'and do you feel nauseous with it'. The GP then names the symptom as 'vertigo' and suggests it is caused by a virus, but states he might come back to it. Later in consultation the GP does come back to the patient's concern.

**Textbox 9.3 Vertigo and drug sheet transcript**

**GP04–02**

```
 1 GP: now you asked a question (that) haven't yet answered which
 2         is (.) whether hydroxychloroquine can cause um vertigo
 3         which I confess I don't know so I'm just going to look it
 4         up ((long inhalation)) (2) however I suspect (.) oh (.) hy-
 5         drox- y (.) I suspect it's um (.) related to the virus
 6         rather [than it's-] jus- it's [(   )      ] timing
 7 PT:         [okay     ]               [but it's-]
 8 PT: so it's not likely to be like (.) the kids used to get
 9         glue ear and that sort of thing that doesn't make you c-
10         have vertigo does it
```

```
11 GP: no n- well in fact it can cause vertigo (.) it's uncommon
12     according to the (.) information sheet but it certainly
13     can
14 PT: mm
15 GP: well there you go (.) you learn something every day
```

At Line 6 the GP invokes the time dimension to suggest that the apparent connection between taking the drug and the unwanted symptom of vertigo is just a coincidence. However, on looking at the drug sheet, he discovers that such a connection is in fact a possibility, and responds fulsomely to the threat to face with 'well there you go (.) you learn something every day' (Line 15). From looking at his other consultations, it is clear that this GP at times uses approaches to diagnosis and treatment that are labelled as complementary and alternative medicine, and this orientation may make him more likely to question prescription medications.

## GP concerns about side effects

GPs may downplay their own or patient concerns about side effects so as to avoid priming patients to pay too much attention to symptoms or out of worry that patients might be dissuaded from taking medications. When they downplay side effects they can use a number of strategies, including using euphemisms, using mitigating language and not responding at all to patient concerns.

Whilst there are certainly a number of instances where GPs do acknowledge and consider options to deal with possible side effects to medication as suggested by patients, the more common response, in our data set at least, is for doctors to contest, downplay or ignore patient-initiated side effects talk. However, it was not uncommon for GPs to raise the issue of side effects when prescribing a new medication or when adjusting one and, more rarely, a GP would associate a patient's symptoms with side effects even when the patient did not. On occasions, GPs could even represent side effects in a positive light – for example, having less energy as a side effect to sleeping pills being represented as a good thing for someone who was overactive.

When GPs initiated side effects talk in relation to a new or changed prescription, a lack of specificity about possible side effects was very common. GPs would use euphemisms, like saying that if a drug is not 'suiting you' other drugs could be tried – what 'not suiting' might mean is often not mentioned. GPs may not elaborate on what the likely side effects are, so the patient may not clearly understand what symptoms could be associated with the medication. One possible reason for euphemistic lexical choice and a lack of specificity is that GPs are avoiding priming the patient to look for certain side effects – GPs may be concerned that doing so would encourage a negative placebo effect. Thus, GPs face a dilemma when raising the issue of side effects: to talk candidly about side effects informs the patient and enhances a genuine process of shared decision-making, but in addition it increases the risk of the prescribed medication having a negative effect on the patient. A further risk, as discussed in Chapter 8, is of discouraging a patient from taking a drug that might be beneficial. Another possible reason for this vague talk is that, as part of their professional working life, it is important for GPs to maintain a particular perspective on medications so that they do not have to continually question their value each time they prescribe, as to do so brings into question the main therapeutic focus of their work.

The following extract illustrates the information asymmetry between patient and doctor in relation to the medications the patient is taking.

---

**Textbox 9.4 What side effects are you expecting transcript**

**TS GP-08-06**

```
 1 PT: could I get um a repeat for the spironolactone while [you]
 2 GP:                                                       [yes]
 3 PT: are there (.)
 4 GP: and (.) how is everything going on that (.) are you still
 5     on one hundred once a day
 6 PT: mmhm
 7 GP: you are quite happy with it
 8 PT: yep its fine
 9 GP: (.) no side effects at all
10 PT: eerrh what side effects are you expecting ha ha I haven't
11     Noticed anything ha ha
12 GP: but you don't get any major diuretic side effects
13 PT: no no
```

---

After the patient's initial denial of any problems (Line 8), the doctor probes further with 'no side effects at all', at which point the patient exhibits a lack of information about possible side effects. This prompts the GP to respond with more detail. If the patient had been told about side effects to the drug in the past she has forgotten, but it seems quite likely that she has never been told, intimated in the patient's phrasing of 'what side effects are you expecting', suggesting that the patient was not expecting any.

With some medications, side effects may be more routinely mentioned, but often in a highly mitigated way such as in the following.

---

**Textbox 9.5 Antibiotics side effects transcript**

**GP02-05**

```
1  GP: there shouldn't be a problem for the antibiotics but
2      occasionally they cause sort of slightly loose bowel
3      motions so er take it with food.
```

---

Here the GP's caution about possible side effects is minimised, with 'sort of slightly' loose motions being presented as an 'occasional' effect, and it is implied that the side effects can be prevented or tempered by the precaution of taking them with food. Providing information about side effects is usually accompanied with the minimising and downgrading of likely effects, which again is perfectly understandable if the GP wants the patient to comply by taking the prescription.

GPs may be more likely to make concerns about side effects explicit in particular situations, for instance, inquiries can readily be made about past side effects when deciding on what medication to prescribe. However, in all instances where discussion of possible future side effects is initiated by the GP, we see the use of mitigators to downgrade the concerns.

The following extract is part of an unusually extensive discussion of side effects. Prior to this sequence, there had already been discussion, initiated by the GP, about the need for caution with painkillers for this particular patient who is on a number of other medications. The specific issue relates to a painful shoulder. This long sequence of side effects talk is most probably a result of the complex medication regime that the patient is on, there being multiple opportunities for adverse interactions between different medications.

---

**Textbox 9.6 Bleed and bleed transcript**

GP07-06

```
 1 GP: your choices for pain killers are (.) you should certainly
 2     be taking panadols (.) two four times a day (.) because
 3     it's (.) it's safe and it (.) will work (.) for at least
 4     part of the pain (.)
 5 PT: m[hm]
 6 GP:  [um] have you got plenty of panadols at ↓home
 7 PT: no no I haven't
 8 GP: right we'll give you a prescription for some cos it's
 9     cheaper if you're using a lot to get it on prescription um
10     (.) the next- you ne- other (.) two other possibilities
11     are codeine which is in the tramadol family but doesn't
12     cost (.) the same amount that tramadol [does        ] (.)
13 PT:                                        [((laughs)) hm]
14 GP: bungs you up a bit (.) um but um (.)otherwise it's a- it's
15     a good pain killer [((inhales))] (.) voltaren (.) um (.)
16 PT.                    [okay      ]
17 GP: tut I can give you um a- a- it's kind of a member of that
18     family that's not quite as hard on the stomach the trouble
19     is with the (.) with the warfarin (.) if you rough up
20     [your] stomach with er an anti inflammatory and it (.) for
21 PT: [yeah]
22 GP: example if you get a stomach ulcer (.) you'll bleed and
23     bleed and bleed and bleed and and it's a bit of a disaster
24     so have to be (.) pretty careful with (.) with voltaren
25     (.) cos all the (.) kind of list of other pills (.)
26     [um so      ] we can either we can either (.) go (.) er
27 PT: [yeah it's ()]
```

```
28 GP: in my- and my feeling is we should probably try and go
29     safely with the one we- that we know is not going to cause
30     any bleeding problems and then if that one doesn't work we
31     can give you the lowest possible dose (.) anti
32     inflammatory that will work I don't mean that you should
33     (.) have horrible pain all the time but we'd try and get a
34     pain killer that (.) kills your pain but (.) doesn't
35 PT: mm hm
36 GP: interact with all the rest of the medicines ((inhales))
37     what do you think
38 PT: (.) ((exhales)) well god (.) I'll try- try anything
39     [to get] (.) er get rid of this
40 GP: [mm    ]
```

In this example the doctor is outlining a number of choices of painkillers that the patient could potentially use and which are commonly prescribed. The GP is explicitly outlining safety concerns in relation to pain relief that works: 'panadol … because it's (.) it's safe and it (.) will work' (Lines 2–3), 'we should probably try and go safely with the one we – that we know is not going to cause any bleeding problems' (Lines 28–30); the Voltaren is potentially dangerous because the patient is on the anticoagulant Warfarin. There is a degree of minimisation and downgrading: 'codeine … bungs you up a bit' (Line 14), another anti-inflammatory may be 'not quite as hard on your stomach' (Line 18). We see extensive upgrading or boosting of both the possible risks from some drugs and the doctor's preferred course of action.

There is an explicit imperative – 'you should certainly be taking panadols' (Lines 1–2); a number of other unqualified assertions – 'it's safe' and 'it will work' (Line 3), 'it's a good pain killer' (Lines 14–15); dramatic word choice – 'disaster' (Line 23), 'rough up your stomach' (Lines 19–20) 'horrible pain all the time' (Line 33); and multiple repetition – 'you'll bleed and bleed and bleed and bleed' (Lines 22–23). Together these create an emphatic effect. The patient's reaction when the doctor asks 'what do you think' in Line 37 suggests he is rather overwhelmed – he exhales and exclaims 'well god' before going on to say he will try anything to get rid of the pain. This example supports the explanation given earlier for why doctors might often avoid such explicit talk about side effects – saying it explicitly may overwhelm the patient with too much information.

The next example illustrates a situation where the GP is considering prescribed medications as a reason for the patient's symptoms of swelling in the legs. In this instance, the patient provides a counter rationale to the GP's suspicions about the medication. The GP asks the patient what medications she is on, and the patient names a number of medications immediately before the following exchange.

The patient here invokes a time dimension to dispute the association of her regular medications with unwanted symptoms (Lines 12–13). This is countered by the GP stating that side effects do not always occur immediately, and 'we

**Textbox 9.7 We don't understand why transcript**

**TSGP08-10**

```
 1 PT: and I mean I'm stabilised on all those medications
 2 GP: yeah
 3 PT: for yonks
 4 GP: yeah
 5 PT: nothing Selena just introduced the bendrofluazide
 6 GP: yeah
 7     ((GP then establishes more detail - lines omitted))
 8 GP: I'm just going to quickly
 9 PT: yeah
10 GP: look up and see if any of these that's a common side
11     effect
12 PT: ohhh okay but surely the fact that I've been on all of
13 PT: [them this time]
14 GP: [well not     ] necessarily you would think
15 PT: yeah
16 GP: Lorna that you would [()and] usually side effects to
17 PT:                       [yeah ]
18 PT: do kick in immediately yeah
19 GP: occur but not always and you can get things
20 PT: yeah
21 GP: and we don't really understand why
22 PT: its just that [pain     ]
23 GP:               [certainly] the um (.) the nardil can which
24     is a common side effect of [that]
25 PT:                            [yeah] but you see I've been on
26     nardil
27 GP: yeah
28 PT: for (.) years
```

don't really understand why' (Lines 14, 16, 19, 21), and that the information he has just looked up (Line 10) suggests that pain is a common side effect of Nardil (Lines 23–24). This line of argument by the GP is in direct contrast to the line of argument used by the GP in the opening transcript of this chapter, suggesting that the 'time' argument is a flexible resource for GPs that can be called upon in different ways to support a particular recommendation or diagnosis. The patient subsequently re-invokes the time dimension – 'yeah but you see I've been on nardil for years' (Lines 25–26) – to cast doubt on the GP's explanation. The statement by the GP here that 'we don't really understand why' is the only instance of such a qualified statement about the state of medical knowledge in relation to side effects talk in this data set (although there are other instances that relate to diagnosis).

In dealing with the medical and interactional dilemmas inherent in side effects talk, GPs can draw on a number of strategies. They can be non-specific in their reference to side effects; they can mitigate or downplay side effects, or suggest preventive action; they can refer to other information, such as the packet inserts, so as to avoid mentioning any specific side effect. The following excerpt illustrates yet another strategy: ignoring the issues raised by a patient. Here the GP initiates a talk about side effects, but does not explicitly respond to the issues raised by the patient at all.

---

**Textbox 9.8 Cold feet transcript**

**GP05-08**

```
 1 GP: and you- do you feel you're having any troubles with
 2     medications
 3 PT: (2) no I mean I still have the cold feet but (.) it's not
 4     bad [um] (2) and=
 5 GP:     [mm]
 6 PT: =sometimes (.) er (.) I get that real er sort of I don't
 7     know (3) I was (.) I don't know whether it's to do with
 8     medication or the blood pressure but (.) for a while I'm-
 9     I've come right again now but it was like in the afternoon
10     having that (.) [absolute] weariness
11 GP:                 [mm      ]
12 GP: mm
13 PT: um but [that-] this last (oh I suppose I've wound up a
14 GP:        [mm   ]
15 PT: bit) but this last week things [haven't] been so bad (.)
16 GP:                                [mm     ]
17 PT: but apart from that nothing really
```

---

Although the GP has made an inquiry about ADRs or 'troubles' (Line 1), when the patient mentions troubles (Lines 3–10), the GP does not attend to them explicitly: the patient's troubles apparently do not align with the troubles that the GP was looking for. As with our first extract in this chapter, the patient presents the troubles in a vague and hesitant way. Her references to 'still' having 'the cold feet' (Line 3), and the statement 'I've come right again now' (Line 9), position her symptoms as not newsworthy, and her subsequent qualifications – 'but (.) it's not bad' (Line 4), 'I don't know whether it's to do with the medication' (Lines 7–8) and 'but this last week things haven't been so bad' (Line 15) – further downplay their significance. The GP listens, but provides only minimal response tokens throughout this presentation, and then turns to the paperwork before handing the patient forms for renewed scripts and terminating the consultation.

## Summing up side effects in the clinic

There are many points we can take from this close analysis of side effects talk in the general practice consultation. One overriding feature is that through this analysis we can discern a mechanism that would more likely lead to an underreporting of side effects than anything else. Primary care physicians in this context are the major clinical contact for the majority of the population, and their primary therapeutic approach is using pharmaceuticals. They also have an important role to play in pharmacovigilance in the post-marketing phase of pharmaceuticals. That is, once pharmaceuticals have come on to the market and passed the requirements of state regulatory agencies, primary care practitioners could act as an important site for reporting of adverse effects. However, our analysis indicates that the clinic is not an ideal site for pharmacovigilance. There are interactional and institutional influences that downplay the chances of side effects being 'recognised' in the primary care consultation, and if they are not recognised they are not reported.

How are we to understand GP behaviour? In general, GPs act to persuade patients to accept and take prescribed medications whilst making them aware of possible side effects. In dealing with this socio-medical dilemma (Heritage and Maynard 2006), GPs tend to use a number of specific discourse strategies, including avoidance, unspecific reference to side effects, and specific references that are downgraded or otherwise qualified. GP presentation of side effects is therefore often vague and general, giving little indication to patients of what they should be looking for.

In addition, GPs may be concerned about the nocebo effect, that is, a negative placebo effect resulting from explicit and specific side effects talk. The extracts on page 126 have illustrated situations where GPs have provided some, if minimal, information about side effects. There are many other consultations where medications are prescribed with no mention of side effects at all. This is less surprising when we consider that to initiate discussion about possible side effects opens up a potential Pandora's Box – where would the GP stop? Given that potentially any drug could cause a range of side effects, addressing all potential concerns could paralyse many consultations.

A more abstract and speculative explanation for GP behaviour, but one that is worth pondering, is that it is an expression of displacement. Emily Martin uses the term displacement to mean 'a social process by which the dangerous parts of an object are removed from direct view' (Martin 2006: 274). GP responses to patient concerns may enact displacement, where the negative and poisonous aspects of medicine are removed from view and the beneficial therapeutic effects stay in focus.

Patients face a different set of concerns when associating symptoms with a prescribed medication. For the patient, to make a claim that a prescribed medication is causing a side effect runs the risk of threatening the therapeutic relationship between doctor and patient. As the GP prescribed the medication that is being claimed to have a negative effect, the claim may threaten the face of the GP, potentially eliciting some uncomfortable emotion like embarrassment or anger if the GP resents the claim. The hedges and qualifiers used by patients can be seen as face-saving work, a way of distancing the patient from any direct criticism of the doctor's prescribing, and so minimising the impact of these face-threatening acts (Brown and Levinson 1987) on both the patient and the doctor.

A few other points are worth mentioning here. One is that using conversation analysis allows the action to be slowed down and scrutinised carefully, and facilitates the observation of processes that people are rarely conscious of. In the case of side effects talk, for example, we can see in action mechanisms that I have described here as face-saving, which have an influence on the outcomes of consultations. It would be difficult to see such mechanisms without a technology like conversation analysis to assist us.

Another point to note is that this research was conducted without any prior idea of what would be found. At the beginning, we simply noted that there was talk about side effects in consultations and that it might be interesting to look at. Once we observed these mechanisms whereby side effects were not acknowledged, we subsequently went to the literature to see what kind of argument we might make of this. It was then that, for me at least, I became aware of the significant underreporting of side effects. So it was with some excitement that I felt that we had found one little piece of the puzzle that would help explain the underreporting of side effects. Because of the interactional dilemmas that are encountered in primary care practice it is not an ideal place to rely on such reporting.

## Concluding comments

Other research had found information on health professionals' and patients' views on these underreporting issues, but had not identified the interactional mechanisms in the way that our research was able to do. For example, other researchers have drawn on interview and survey data to conclude that health professionals underreport ADRs for many reasons including a lack of awareness of the kinds of reactions that need reporting, concern about reporting only suspected ADRs and a view that only safe drugs are released to the market (Lopez-Gonzalez *et al.* 2009). Additionally, there is a reluctance to report ADRs if the reaction was not well-known, due to a lack of knowledge of existing reporting rules and due to a lack of time (Backstrom *et al.* 2000).

ADRs reported by patients are consistently dismissed by health professionals, even those that are well-documented (Pound *et al.* 2005). For example, when patients complained about muscle aches, pain, memory lapses or cognitive impairments from taking statins, half of them had their concerns dismissed by physicians (Light 2010). Another interview-based study (Britten *et al.* 2004) found that most patients attending general practice consultations expressed an aversion to medications. Those interviewed also had consultations with their GP recorded, and it was found that there were no cases where there was a 'genuine discussion' of the patients' views, and that patients tended to express their aversion to medicines in the consultation in a muted fashion (Britten *et al.* 2004). Nicky Britten and colleagues (Britten *et al.* 2004) argue that there is a need for a 'culture shift' so that patients can express their aversion to medicines. GPs may be able to foster such a shift by taking patients' claims at face value as being worthy of investigation, but this is not a straightforward matter as it would add layers of complexity to the consultation.

In a Swedish study of 51 doctor-patient consultations about antihypertensive medication, 21 patients talked in the consultation about the effects of medication, mainly unwanted reactions or side effects (Kjellgren *et al.* 1998). In interviews, 20 out of 33 patients reported side effects from their current antihypertensive medication (Kjellgren *et al.* 1998). However, the authors note that side effects as a term was seldom used by either patients or physicians. In an observation study related to antipsychotic medication consultations, patient concerns about ADRs would commonly receive no response from the psychiatrist, or the psychiatrist would change the subject or disagree with the patient's interpretation (Seale *et al.* 2007). That is, there is a growing literature that aligns with our findings.

The kind of 'displacement' we see in these consultations is an important feature of pharmaceuticalised governance. It indicates interactional features that occur in the consultation that shape decision-making and medication practices. Patients are constrained and prescribers of medications conduct themselves in particular ways. In the clinical space we can observe interactional mechanisms that promote conformity to medication practices and downgrade concerns about medications. I suggest that this aspect of governance is not driven by profit motives, but is an outcome of complex everyday interactions in health care settings.

A number of years after this research was completed (although at one level research is very often never completed), I embarked on some other research, again in an 'inductive way', which gave me further insight into this underreporting issue. This research was on a pharmaceutical controversy, the case of Eltroxin in New Zealand, and the following chapter will address this case.

## Appendix

The following are the transcription conventions used in some of the transcripts.

```
(.)            denotes a micro-pause
(2)            denotes a pause of the specified number of
seconds
[ ]            denotes overlapping talk
(and)          words in single parentheses denote
               candidate hearings
Certainly      underlined word denotes increased emphasis
=              denotes latching or no gap between talk
((laughs))     words in double parentheses denotes
               descriptions that have been added by the
               author
GP:            refers to the general practitioner
               speaking
PT:            refers to the patient speaking
```

## References

Backstrom, M., Mjorndal, T., Dahlqvist, R. and Nordkvist-Olsson, T. (2000). Attitudes to reporting adverse drug reactions in northern Sweden. *European Journal of Clinical Pharmacology* 56 (9–10): 729–732.

Britten, N., Stevenson, F., Gafaranga, J., Barry, C. and Bradley, C. (2004). The expression of aversion to medicines in general practice consultations. *Social Science and Medicine* 59: 1495–1503.

Brown, P. and Levinson, S. (1987). *Politeness: Some Universals in Language Usage.* Cambridge: Cambridge University Press.

Dew, K., Stubbe, M., Macdonald, L. and Dowell, A. (2012). Side effects talk in general practice consultations. In: *Medical Communication in Clinical Contexts* (eds B. Bates and R. Ahmed), 95–126. Dubuque IA: Kendall Hunt.

Dew, K., Stubbe, M., Macdonald, L., Dowell, A. and Plumridge, E. (2010). The (non) use of prioritisation protocols by surgeons. *Sociology of Health and Illness* 32 (4): 545–562.

Gill, V. and Maynard, D.W. (2006). Explaining illness: Patients' proposals and physician' responses. In: *Communication in Medical Care: Interaction Between Primary Care Physicians and Patients* (eds J. Heritage and D.W. Maynard), 115–150. Cambridge: Cambridge University Press.

Goffman, E. (1967). *Interaction Ritual: Essays on Face-To-Face Behaviour.* Harmondsworth: Penguin.

Hazell, L. and Shakir, S.A.W. (2006). Under-reporting of adverse drug reactions: A systematic review. *Drug Safety* 29 (5): 385–396.

Heritage, J. and Maynard, D.W. (2006). Introduction. In: *Communication in Medical Care: Interaction Between Primary Care Physicians and Patients* (eds J. Heritage and D.W. Maynard). Cambridge: Cambridge University Press.

Kjellgren, K.I., Svensson, S., Ahlner, J. and Saljo, R. (1998). Antihypertensive medication in clinical encounters. *International Journal of Cardiology* 64 (2): 161–169.

Light, D. (2010). Bearing the risks of prescription drugs. In: *The Risks of Prescription Drugs* (ed. D. Light), 1–39. New York: Columbia University Press.

Lopez-Gonzalez, E., Herdeiro, M.T. and Figueiras, A. (2009). Determinants of underreporting of adverse drug reactions: A systematic review. *Drug Safety* 32 (1): 19–31.

Manning, P. (1992). *Erving Goffman and Modern Sociology.* Stanford: Stanford University Press.

Martin, E. (2006). The pharmaceutical person. *BioSocieties* 1 (3): 273–287.

Pound, P., Britten, N., Morgan, M., Yardley, L., Pope, C., Daker-White, G. and Campbell, R. (2005). Resisting medicine: A synthesis of qualitative studies of medicine taking. *Social Science and Medicine* 61: 133–155.

Schegloff, E., Jefferson, G. and Sacks, H. (1977). The preference for self-correction in the organization of repair in conversation. *Language* 53 (2): 361–382.

Seale, C., Chaplin, R., Lelliot, P. and Quirk, A. (2007). Antipsychotic medication, sedation and mental clouding: An observational study of psychiatric consultations. *Social Science and Medicine* 65 (4): 698–711.

Spelsberg, A., Prugger, C., Doshi, P., Ostrowski, K., Witte, T., Husgen, D. and Keil, U. (2017). Contribution of industry funded post-marketing studies to drug safety: Survey of notifications submitted to regulatory agencies. *British Medical Journal* 356: j337.

# 10 Pharmacovigilance lessons

The study of Eltroxin was the outcome of a different research process from the one described in the previous chapter. In this instance, I was involved in research with a number of colleagues looking at how people used medications in the home, a project we referred to as the social meanings of medication research, noted in Chapter 4. As part of that research we wanted to look at some drug-based controversies reported in the media, to see if we could identify if and how such reporting impacted upon our research participants. One example we looked at was Herceptin: we explored the processes leading to the decision of the New Zealand government to fund this particular anti-cancer drug despite the decision not being supported by its own regulatory agency (Gabe *et al.* 2012). More on this in the following chapter. The example of Eltroxin, however, came to have a more direct bearing on the issue of underreporting of side effects.

This piece of research came about after one of my research team colleagues, Pauline Norris, had a discussion with a member of the Centre for Adverse Reactions Monitoring (CARM) team based at the University of Otago in Dunedin, New Zealand. CARM staff were puzzled by a sudden spike in reports of adverse reactions to a drug used to treat hypothyroidism, Eltroxin and were interested in obtaining some perspectives on this from social scientists.

New Zealand has a public health system where approved drugs are government subsidised. The agency responsible for regulating therapeutic products in New Zealand and overseeing pharmacovigilance activities is Medsafe (the New Zealand Medicines and Medical Devices Safety Authority, a business unit of the Ministry of Health), and responsibility for approving medications to be listed for subsidy rests with PHARMAC (the Pharmaceutical Management Agency). The New Zealand Pharmacovigilance Centre (NZPVC) is responsible for post-marketing surveillance of medications. CARM is part of the NZPVC, and relies on a spontaneous reporting scheme for identifying adverse reactions. That is, it does not proactively seek out information about adverse reactions, but relies on patients and health professionals to make reports to CARM. The Medicines Adverse Reactions Committee (MARC) acts as an independent advisory committee to the Ministry of Health, and committee members are practising medical practitioners. MARC receives material from CARM and other sources, and acts as an advisor to Medsafe.

In July 2007, a new formulation of Eltroxin, the drug subsidised by PHARMAC to treat hypothyroidism, was introduced into New Zealand and 70,000 people with hypothyroidism were phased onto the new formulation. This new formulation was a result of the manufacturer, GlaxoSmithKline, consolidating its manufacturing operations. The active ingredient was not changed, but the tablet was changed from a yellow colour to white. Prior to the formulation change, CARM had received about one report every two to three years where thyroxine was the suspect agent, coming to a total of 14 reports of adverse drug reactions (ADRs) to thyroxine medications between 1973 and 2007. CARM received the first report of a problem attributed to the new formulation on 8 October 2007. After the formulation change occurred, reports of adverse reactions began to appear in the media. The new formulation was linked by various users to a range of adverse effects from joint and muscle pain, weight gain and depression, to conjunctivitis, skin rash and visual disturbances. Despite assurances from both the drug manufacturer and Medsafe that the new formulation was safe for use, reports of adverse reactions continued to accumulate, with over 800 ADRs reported by September 2008 (Gardner and Dew 2011).

I travelled to Dunedin to talk to the people at CARM to get a sense of this. CARM were genuinely puzzled. To their understanding, the new formulation of Eltroxin was no different in terms of its toxicity or therapeutic efficacy to the old formulation. In other words, it was thought to be bioequivalent. Another group of researchers had expressed interest in this issue to CARM, and provided a very particular interpretation of this event, putting it down to an irrational response from vulnerable patients (Faasse *et al.* 2010), which I will return to shortly. I was perhaps alerted to this type of interpretation when I first discussed this issue with my research team. At a team meeting, I noted the puzzle that was set before us, but the immediate response from some of my colleagues was that the excess reporting would be a result of social contagion or mass hysteria. At the time I pointed out that we had no evidence of this and that we should not presume the outcome of our research before we started it. My colleagues agreed with me on this point.

In trying to get some understanding of this puzzle I was lucky enough to have John Gardner come on board to help out with the research; John had recently completed a superb Master's thesis and I was delighted that this puzzle piqued his interest. John set to work collecting data from relevant media, predominantly newspapers, from the period of the controversy, June 2008 to August 2009. Press releases from PHARMAC, Medsafe, the Ministry of Health and political parties were obtained, as were the minutes from MARC meetings that reviewed Eltroxin. John's initial approach to this data was to identify the sequence of events, the different actors involved and how these actors responded to the controversy, drawing on an Actor-Network-Theory orientation. By using this approach we were able to focus on what actors emerged as the controversy unfolded, how they defined the debate and how the controversy was resolved (Dew *et al.* 2017; Gardner and Dew 2011).

## Eltroxin events

I will briefly summarise the unfolding of events. The link between the new Eltroxin formulation and a series of reported ADRs was first publicised a year after the introduction of the new formulation by a regional newspaper, *The Southland Times*, which provided patients' accounts of adverse reactions after the switch to the new formulation. Later newspaper articles elaborated on the alternative medication that patients claimed did not cause adverse reactions, levothyroxine manufactured by Goldshield Ltd. (Gerken 2008a). However, this formulation was not subsidised by PHARMAC, requiring patients to pay the full cost of the medication. A later article in the same paper reported that CARM wanted to hear from people who had experienced side effects to Eltroxin, and provided instructions on how to contact CARM at the end of the article (Gerken 2008c). By providing these instructions the media opened up a channel for Eltroxin users to contact CARM directly. Although direct patient reporting to CARM was already a possibility, it is unlikely that patients were aware CARM existed or, if they were, they may not have realised that they could make reports directly to CARM. To illustrate, there are pamphlets on adverse reactions to vaccines that can be displayed in general practitioner (GP) waiting rooms that mention CARM, but these pamphlets state that patients should inform their GPs about any reactions, and these pamphlets provide no information on how to access CARM directly. I have tested this out regularly in the sociology of health and illness classes I teach: I ask students if they have heard of CARM or if they knew how to report adverse reactions to drugs, but am yet to find someone who knows.

After this initial coverage by *The Southland Times*, media coverage spread to other parts of the country. Around this time, Medsafe issued a press release stating that they were satisfied with the safety and quality of the drug's new formulation, and suggesting that 'poor patient compliance should be considered as a possible cause of adverse effects' (Medsafe 2008). That is, the source of the problem was being identified as the patient who, with the new formulation, started to non-comply in ways that they never did before. It is difficult to see how such a claim would be arrived at. What is it about the new formulation that would suddenly make the compliant patient non-compliant? Following this, members of parliament got involved in the controversy, and in their press releases they again provided information on how to contact CARM. There were questions in parliament and more media coverage ramping up concerns about the drug. MARC discussed the concerns, noting that on October 2007 there were only 14 reports or ADRs received for the drug but by September 2008 this had increased to 810 reports, with 40 per cent of those made directly by patients. Typically patients only make up 1–2 per cent of reports (MARC 2008) – usually, nearly all reports are made by health professionals. Three types of symptoms were most commonly described: hypothyroid-type symptoms (53 per cent); headache (29 per cent) and hypersensitivity (28 per cent).

The Pharmacovigilance Centre contacted 83 countries on the World Health Organization's adverse reactions monitoring scheme. There had been no reports of adverse reactions to the new GlaxoSmithKline formulation, although similar adverse reactions had been reported in some countries to other brands of thyroxine. After considering the reports of both CARM and Medsafe, MARC concluded that there was no 'specific medical, physiological or pharmacological explanation for the increase in adverse reaction reports' (MARC 2008). But it noted that reports of improvement after switching brands added weight to the argument that there may be some link. If a different brand relieved symptoms perhaps the new formulation was having some physiological effect.

Many patients were turning to Goldshield as a better alternative, even though it could only be purchased at the unsubsidised price. According to an article in *The Press*, the company responsible for supplying the unsubsidised drug to New Zealand could not obtain enough supplies to keep up with demand (Wylie 2008). Pharmacists' directly imported stocks of other unsubsidised drugs such as levothyroxine (Goldshield) manufactured in the United Kingdom and Synthroid (levothyroxine, Abbott Laboratories) manufactured in Canada (Gerken 2008b). By the end of September 2008, PHARMAC made the decision to subsidise Goldshield for those who were intolerant to the new Eltroxin formulation (PHARMAC 2008). After the introduction of the new subsidised Goldshield, media coverage quickly became much less frequent, as did reporting of ADRs.

## Explanations for the ADRs

As mentioned, following these events another research team attempted to come to some understanding of what turned out to be a more than 400-fold increase in patient-reported ADRs for Eltroxin in New Zealand. The conclusion this research team came to was essentially the same as the one my colleagues had initially suggested was likely. Faasse and colleagues suggested that the increase in reported ADRs was a likely result of an irrational response from hypothyroid patients, where media coverage, distrust of PHARMAC, and the agitation of a few key individuals encouraged a group of patients prone to emotional distress to attribute their various health problems to the new drug formulation (Faasse *et al.* 2010; Faasse *et al.* 2012). This kind of argument allows a business-as-usual approach to pharmacovigilance. It assumes that the current level of reporting of ADRs is appropriate, and therefore any excess needs to be explained away. A simple explanation is that it is the result of people being irrational. This explanation was simply an assertion. No evidence was produced to support it and no testing was undertaken to determine if people were being irrational, or if they were prone to emotional responses. It is simply an assertion, based on the possibility that people with thyroid conditions might be emotionally vulnerable. The assertion was a powerful one, with the article appearing in the well-read and highly respected *British Medical Journal*. When we approached the same clinical journal with our different explanation, based on a closer analysis of the actual unfolding of events, we were declined that opportunity to publish. One possible reason for this rejection is that the narrative provided by Faasse and colleagues allows for the simple restoration of normality: the case can be closed and nothing more needs to be done about it, because we cannot control for irrational individuals. There has been a tradition of dismissing patient reports of safety problems with medicines, which has thus, further exposed people to unsafe products (Abraham and Shepherd 1999; Mintz 1985).

Another possible explanation for the increase in ADRs is that the assumptions of the drug safety regulators were in error. There is some evidence to support this explanation. Medsafe accepted that bioequivalence fell within an internationally accepted range (Medsafe 2010). However, this range for thyroid medication is not accepted in every jurisdiction. In a joint statement the American Thyroid Association, The Endocrine Society, and American Association of Clinical Endocrinologists argue that 'levothyroxine is a drug recognized to have a narrow toxic to therapeutic ratio with significant clinical consequences of excessive or inadequate treatment' (American Thyroid Association *et al.* 2004). So, although the view in New Zealand was that the new formulation of Eltroxin was bioequivalent to the previous formulation, the 80–125 per cent range of bioequivalence that it used is broad compared to the narrow toxic to therapeutic ratio of the medication. Further, a survey of American physicians prescribing thyroxine found that switching between approved preparations was associated with some adverse outcomes, frequently resulting from generic substitution without the prescriber's knowledge (Hennessey *et al.* 2010). Switching between thyroxine-containing products can usually be managed to avoid adverse reactions by readjusting the dosage. However, for CARM switching products may have led to a short-term increase in reported ADRs during the phase of dose adjustment, that is, during the phase when clinicians would adjust the amount prescribed in response to patient symptoms. In the New Zealand context, because PHARMAC only subsidised the one formulation it was not so easy for clinicians to prescribe a different brand, even if another brand was available, because the patients would have to pay the full price.

Another piece of the puzzle is the new ADR reporting mechanism that opened up during the Eltroxin media coverage, through which the usual institutionalised processes of reporting, primarily undertaken through the GP, was considerably augmented. When I started thinking about this, I had what some have called an 'aha' moment. I was now able to link this research with my earlier research on side effects talk in the consultation. It seemed obvious to me now what was happening. The standard form of reporting meant likely underreporting, because the interactional and clinical requirements of the GP consultation did not facilitate the process. We had seen how this worked in practice. Now, in the media coverage of Eltroxin, patients were explicitly asked to contact CARM about ADRs directly, and they did. From this perspective, the Eltroxin controversy did not constitute an over-reporting of adverse reactions, but rather allowed for an enhanced level of reporting and registering of patient concerns. The media played an important role in this, by providing the information about contacting CARM and alerting patients to the possibility that what they were experiencing could be the result of the medication they were on. This important role of the media is well noted in the scholarly literature (Gabe and Bury 1996; Hooker

2010). Figure 10.1 graphically illustrates the different processes of reporting of Eltroxin compared to usual processes of reporting.

Under the 'Usual Process', GPs and other health professionals are the typical source of ADR reports in New Zealand. However, there are several barriers to reporting with this mechanism. First, the patient has to consider his or her symptom to be a result of the prescribed medication. This connection could be particularly difficult to make, especially for people with co-morbidities or chronic illness where symptoms fluctuate. This issue was reinforced for me when I undertook interviews of householders for another arm of this research into the social meanings of medications. In one of the households that I went to, one person had a diagnosis of hypothyroidism and was on Eltroxin. In her inter-view, which was undertaken with her husband as well, she recounted the follow-ing in relation to being switched to the new Eltroxin formulation:

> Yeah, like headaches and my blurry eyes. I went to the optician thinking maybe my eyes, I needed new glasses. And I was sort of getting headaches and what was the other thing I was getting? I can't remember. Oh, aching muscles. Remember my leg muscles were getting, like, really achy in the mornings. Particularly when I got up, like, as though you had no power in your legs. And all that sort of thing and I never put, never thought about that drug.

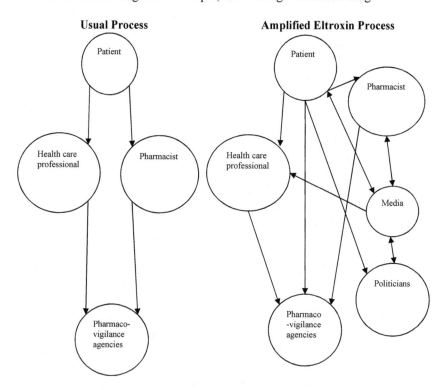

*Figure 10.1* Processes of alerting to adverse reactions in New Zealand.

She went on to say:

> I had a lot of problems and I, then I heard them talking on the Talkback about people with the same problems and I thought, 'Well, that's strange, that's the sort of thing I've been having'. But because I was on quite a bit of other medication I sort of thought, 'Well, maybe it was just something to do with that'. And that's when I went back to the pharmacist first and said, 'Can I go back onto Eltroxin that I was originally taking?'. He said, 'Well, no, because they're not bringing it into the country', or something now. So I made a note in my diary about what I'd heard and that there was Gold-Shield. So then I went to my GP and I said I wasn't happy about the stuff that I was taking and could I try the GoldShield and he was quite happy to do that. So I switched to the GoldShield.

Far from being irrational, the participant went through a process of considering a number of competing explanations for her new symptoms before pushing for a switch to her medication. The media again played an important role, in this case making available information that allowed her to consider another explanation for her new symptoms. It is, however, unlikely that her symptoms were reported to CARM, as the problem had been resolved with the subsidisation of other brands.

Another barrier for patients is that they have to confront the health professional, usually their GP, with the bad news that a prescribed medication is causing problems. As I noted in the previous chapter, this is a face-threatening act – it threatens the face of the health professional – and so patients may be reluctant to raise the issue of side effects. However, now that concerns about Eltroxin were more widely available, the threat to face may have been substantially lowered.

The augmented Eltroxin Process of ADR reporting is shown in the right side of Figure 10.1 (Amplified Eltroxin Process). With media involvement, patients who read or hear media reports can now potentially relate their symptoms to the medication they are taking, possibly helping to overcome the first barrier mentioned on page 140. Further, GPs and other health professionals may, due to the media coverage, become more aware of the possibility that symptoms the patient presents with are a result of a medication. Politicians can be alerted by patients directly or through media coverage and in turn facilitate further coverage. Cumulatively, these processes can have at least two consequences: first, GPs may be more likely to take a patient's association of symptoms with the medication as a real possibility, and second, GPs may themselves make the connection between a patient's symptoms and their medication without the patient making that connection. This provides more opportunities for associations to be made and ADRs to be reported.

We can still anticipate underreporting here: even if patients associate symptoms with the medication, they still may not wish to threaten the face of the health professional. However, with the media providing details about who to report ADRs to, patients can go directly to CARM and bypass the health professional thus, avoiding the face-threatening act. This is precisely what occurred in the Eltroxin controversy, with CARM receiving an unusually high number of reports directly from patients. Although it was always possible for patients to report ADRs directly to CARM, they were unaware of this opportunity, and it had not previously been utilised. With the extensive media coverage of the controversy alerting people to CARM, it is little wonder that there were higher rates of ADR reports.

The role of PHARMAC is undoubtedly important in the playing out of this controversy as well. As PHARMAC initially subsidised only Eltroxin and no other brands, it was less likely that patients would switch to other medications to treat hypothyroidism, as they would have had to pay the full, unsubsidised cost and supplies of such drugs were limited. This meant that media could only describe the problem, and not offer solutions to patients except the possibility of paying for the unsubsidised medications if they were available at local pharmacies. In other countries where the new formulation was introduced, such as Germany and the Netherlands, alternative brands were available and no significant increases in ADRs occurred (MARC 2008). With other brands available patients could readily switch medications without the need to report. In effect, there was no 'release valve' to divert concerns about ADRs in New Zealand as there was in other jurisdictions where the new formula was used.

The case of Eltroxin provides important insights into ADR underreporting. It suggests that there needs to be more effort put into opening up reporting channels, and given the high level of underreporting we should perhaps be less concerned with trying to explain any increase in reporting levels as a psychological problem residing with the drug users.

## Enhancing pharmacovigilance

An important issue we can take from this case study of Eltroxin is that, if we are concerned about the underreporting of side effects, we need to more vigilantly deploy other means of promoting such reporting that does not rely on the health professionals who prescribe the medication. Indeed, there is much endeavour going into this. But before considering some of those, it is worth noting that the reception of the argument I have presented here has had a troubled path at times. I mention this because again it suggests how normality, or business-as-usual, can be preserved, at least in academic circles. I have already mentioned the lack of interest in this version of events from the *British Medical Journal*, even though the journal had published an alternative version based on assertion and little evidence. Later, an article based on this research was sent to a well-known social science journal, *Social Science and Medicine*. The editor who looked at the article refused to send it out to review, on the basis that the argument we were making in the article was normative. Indeed it was normative, in the sense that, if we are concerned about underreporting, then we ought to do something. The 'ought' in that last sentence is considered by some to be normative. But, of course, an accusation of being normative is close to an absurdity. It is impossible to avoid being normative. To illustrate this simply – rejecting an article because it 'ought' to avoid being normative is being normative.

There are attempts made around the world to enhance pharmacovigilance. Many countries, including New Zealand, operate under a largely passive pharmacovigilance system. That is, the different agencies responsible for drug safety assess reports that come in about side effects of drugs on the market, but they do not actively seek to identify or generate reports of side effects. There are more active pharmacovigilance surveillance systems, such as those in the United States (US), which actively look at patient records to detect post-marketing concerns about ADRs (Wiktorowicz *et al.* 2012). In the Netherlands, websites have been created specifically for reporting by patients. Other mechanisms to encourage patient exchange of information could be considered, for example, online patient support forums allowing patients to tell their own medication stories (Knezevic *et al.* 2011; Medawar *et al.* 2002). By reading the stories of others, patients can consider the validity of their own stories. Drug safety agencies could actively monitor these sites to see if there are any issues that could be followed up. Patients should be made aware of such sites, with information about them provided by those who prescribe the medication. In the US the Food and Drug Administration Amendments Act (FDAAA) of 2007 mandated that printed direct-to-consumer advertisements for prescription drugs include the following statement presented in conspicuous text: 'You are encouraged to report negative side effects of prescription drugs to the FDA. Visit www.fda.gov/medwatch, or call 1-800-FDA-1088'.

Media is another channel for promoting enhanced ADR reporting, particularly in a passive reporting environment. Stories circulated through news media can establish other opportunities for reporting, such as the establishment of patient support groups and websites, and they can facilitate discussions of ADRs in patient-doctor interactions. For example, Charles Medawar and colleagues note that television publicity associated with Seroxat (paroxetine) contributed to many user reports about the drug effects being posted on websites. Many users stated that prior to seeing the comments of others on these websites, they had not associated their symptoms with the medications in question (Medawar *et al.* 2002). In the case of Eltroxin, support groups and websites were established. Additionally, regional newspapers played an important role in disseminating information. There is potential here for pharmacovigilance agencies to make more use of smaller regional newspapers, often more eager to have news stories, to publicise concerns and raise their own profiles.

I suggest that it is important to consider these alternative reporting strategies given opposing tendencies that limit reporting once drugs come on to the market. Chapter 8 noted some of the limitations and concerns raised around pre-clinical trials of pharmaceuticals. Concerns have similarly been raised about how pharmaceutical companies shape research and knowledge production in the post-marketing phase of newly approved pharmaceuticals. Research suggests that the underreporting of adverse reactions to drugs may be made worse by post-marketing trials that are supposed to enhance pharmacovigilance. This is simply achieved by enrolling prescribing physicians into post-marketing trials. In this situation, physicians are highly remunerated for their participation. By providing the drug to their patients as part of the trial, drug companies may get a competitive edge over their rivals. In these trials the enrolled physicians may sign up to confidentiality clauses that prevent them from reporting any adverse reactions to pharmacovigilance agencies. Research undertaken by Spelsberg and colleagues (2017) in Germany elucidate this process.

In Germany, legislation on medicinal products requires drug companies to register any post-marketing studies undertaken by the drug company. Germany is the only country with such a law (Spelsberg *et al.* 2017). Drug companies register their trials with three authorities: the Statutory Health Insurance authority, the National Association of Statutory Health Insurance Physicians and the drug regulator. Germany thus, has a repository of information on post-marketing trials of drugs. However, accessing such information is not straightforward. These agencies are theoretically independent of the drug companies, but nevertheless, when Spelsberg and colleagues made freedom of information requests, the agencies withheld information on various grounds, including concerns about protecting the confidentiality and business secrets of the companies (Spelsberg *et al.* 2017). These agencies exhibit what John Abraham refers to as corporate bias, working to protect the business interests of drug companies.

Spelsberg and colleagues had to successfully sue one registration authority in order to gain access to the information. Once they obtained this access, they were able to identify the amount of remuneration that physicians were paid for participating in post-marketing trials, with some earning more than €200,000 per study. Physicians signed confidentiality agreements, which included keeping the results of the study confidential. The confidentiality agreement meant that any adverse reactions could be reported only to the sponsor of the trial and not to pharmacovigilance agencies, thus even further enhancing physician under-reporting of adverse events. So in these post-marketing trials there is an increase in prescribing of a drug because physicians are being paid to do so, and a decrease in reporting of any adverse reactions because those physicians are contractually bound not to report them. In addition, Spelsberg and colleagues found that most of the study designs for the trials were very limited, for example, not having comparison groups and enrolling small numbers of participants, making it impossible to interpret the results in any meaningful way. Such scenarios can easily undermine post-marketing pharmacovigilance efforts.

In the case of post-marketing trials we see another dilemma at play. On the one hand physicians are encouraged to report adverse reactions to drugs, and on the other hand they are held to account to maintain the commercial interests of drug companies. What is pitched as important post-marketing surveillance activities is undertaken for commercial gain.

## Concluding comments

Given the limitations of scientific trials and the strategies of drug companies, the reporting of ADRs when drugs are on the market would appear to be an important drug safety measure. This reporting can happen at a variety of inter-related levels, through both official and informal channels. These involve patients reporting to doctors, doctors reporting to pharmacovigilance systems, patients reporting to patients through conversations and social networking, and patients reporting to journalists in news media stories. There are, however, many influences that work against pharmacovigilance activities: the work of drug companies to keep their drugs on the market; the difficulties of having ADRs recognised in clinical consultations; the efforts of academics and experts to explain away ADR reports.

Years after we had completed our research on the Eltroxin case another drug company, Merck, changed its formulation of thyroxine used to treat hypothyroid patients. In France in 2017, thousands of patients who went on the new formulation complained about side effects, and other countries including the US, China and Brazil requested a return to the old formulation (Sciama 2017). The New Zealand experience was repeated.

Pharmacovigilance, or the lack of it, is an important aspect of pharmaceuticalised governance. Poor vigilance provides drug prescribers and users with distorted information. It is more likely that patients will suffer from symptoms that are caused by drugs, but neither the health professionals nor the patients are able to make that association. Symptoms are explained away, or put down to other causes. On the other hand, to enhance pharmacovigilance may require embracing drug users' claims of possible problems with drugs. Endeavours to improve pharmacovigilance may enhance patient self-monitoring, which in turn may promote anxiety. Furthermore, increasing levels of pharmacovigilance may require more effort from drug safety agencies, drug prescribers and drug users to resist drug company attempts to downplay concerns about ADRs. Chapter 12 turns to a broader discussion of resistance to pharmaceuticalised governance.

## References

Abraham, J. and Shepherd, J. (1999). *The Therapeutic Nightmare: The Battle Over the World's Most Controversial Sleeping Pill.* Abingdon: Earthscan.

American Thyroid Association, The Endocrine Society and American Association of Clinical Endocrinologists. (2004). Joint statement on the U.S. Food and Drug Administration's decision regarding bioequivalence of levothyroxine sodium. *Thyroid* 14 (7): 486.

Dew, K., Gardner, J., Morrato, E., Norris, P., Chamberlain, K., Hodgetts, D. and Gabe, J. (2017). Public engagement and the role of the media in post-marketing drug safety: The case of Eltroxin® (levothyroxine) in New Zealand. *Critical Public Health* 1–14. doi:10.1080/09581596.2017.1329520.

Faasse, K., Cundy, T. and Petrie, K. (2010). Thyroxine: Anatomy of a health scare. *British Medical Journal* 340: 20–21.

Faasse, K., Gamble, G., Cundy, T. and Petrie, K. (2012). Impact of television coverage on the number and type of symptoms reported during a health scare: A retrospective pre–post observational study. *BMJ Open* 2: e001607.

Gabe, J. and Bury, M. (1996). Halcion nights: A sociological account of a medical controversy. *Sociology* 30 (3): 447–469.

Gabe, J., Chamberlain, K., Norris, P., Dew, K., Madden, H. and Hodgettse, D. (2012). The debate about the funding of Herceptin: A case study of 'countervailing powers'. *Social Science and Medicine* 75 (12): 2353–2361.

Gardner, J. and Dew, K. (2011). The Eltroxin controversy: Risk and how actors construct their world. *Health, Risk and Society* 13 (5): 397–411.

Gerken, S. (2008a). Changes to thyroid drug formula blamed for sickness. *The Southland Times* (7 June).

Gerken, S. (2008b). Huge demand for alternative drug. *The Southland Times* (23 September).

Gerken, S. (2008c). Thyroid drug users urged to contact centre. *The Southland Times* (14 June).

Hennessey, J., Malabanan, A., Haugen, B. and Levy, E. (2010). Adverse event reporting in patients treated with Levothyroxine: Results of the Pharmacovigilance Task Force survey of the American Thyroid Association, American Association of Clinical Endocrinologists and The Endocrine Society. *Endocrine Practice* 16 (3): 357–370.

Hooker, C. (2010). Health scares: Professional priorities. *Health* 14 (1): 3–21.

Knezevic, M., Bivolarevic, I., Peric, T. and Jankovic, S. (2011). Using Facebook to increase spontaneous reporting of adverse drug reactions. *Drug Safety* 34 (4): 351–352.

MARC. (2008). *Minutes of 135th Meeting Held on 11 September 2008*. Wellington: Medicines Adverse Reactions Monitoring Committee.

Medawar, C., Herxheimer, A., Bell, A. and Jofre, S. (2002). Paroxetine, panorama and user reporting of ADRs: Consumer intelligence matters in clinical practice and post-marketing drug surveillance. *International Journal of Risk and Safety in Medicine* 15: 161–169.

Medsafe. (2008). Press release: Eltroxin formulation change. *Scoop Media Limited* (27 June).

Medsafe. (2010). Eltroxin formulation change. www.medsafe.govt.nz/hot/alerts/Eltroxin-Info.asp (accessed 3 September 2010). Wellington: Medsafe.

Mintz, M. (1985). *At Any Cost: Corporate Greed, Women, and the Dalkon Shield.* New York: Pantheon Books.

PHARMAC. (2008). Press release: Consultation on alternative thyroid treatment. *Scoop Media Limited* (30 September).

Sciama, Y. (2017). France brings back a phased-out drug after patients rebel against its replacement. *Science* (27 Sept). doi:10.1126/science.aaq0705.

Spelsberg, A., Prugger, C., Doshi, P., Ostrowski, K., Witte, T., Husgen, D. and Keil, U. (2017). Contribution of industry funded post-marketing studies to drug safety: survey of notifications submitted to regulatory agencies. *British Medical Journal* 356: j337.

Wiktorowicz, M., Lexchin, J. and Moscou, K. (2012). Pharmacovigilance in Europe and North America: Divergent approaches. *Social Science and Medicine* 75: 165–170.

Wylie, K. (2008). Alternative drug sells out. *The Press* (29 August).

# 11 Different faces of governance

This chapter explores some of the ways that social organisation shapes drug development and drug consumption. However, rather than considering this as a one way development, that is, social organisation does the determining, I want to highlight in this chapter how drug development and consumption shape the social world. I consider some ways in which people, states and pharmaceuticals interact over time and in different locales. Pharmaceuticalised governance takes many different forms. It is shaped by the particular social and cultural setting in which pharmaceuticals are developed, prescribed, purchased and used. In turn, pharmaceuticals play, at least in my reading, an extraordinary role in shaping societies and cultures, from the way they are emphasised by states as solutions to problems, to their ability to transform identities and relationships between people. Drug companies develop particular strategies to shape pharmaceuticalised governance, and people, corporations and states may use pharmaceuticals to mediate other forms of governance, that is, to bring about changes in social organisation and social interaction.

In this chapter, I open up the debate by noting the diversity in consumption patterns of pharmaceuticals across nation-states. The case of antibiotic consumption, used here to illustrate these differences in consumption, suggest that there is something quite nationally specific about the relationship between forms of social organisation and drug consumption. In the rest of the chapter, I reflect on some contrasts between the Global North and the Global South in their relationships to pharmaceuticals, considering issues of drug development and financing, the targets of drug company strategies and some ways in which the same pharmaceutical interventions can have very different outcomes for those in different parts of the global economy.

## Diverse consumption patterns

Tanja Mueller and Per-Olof Östergren describe different patterns of antibiotic consumption in the European Union. The case of antibiotic consumption is insightful, given concerns about over prescribing and inappropriate antibiotic use. Whereas pharmaceuticals were once seen as capable of bringing about the demise of infectious diseases, there are now increasing concerns about resistance to antibiotics and apocalyptic predictions of cleverly mutating microbes signalling a new post-antibiotic era (Brown and Crawford 2009). Particular concerns have been raised over multidrug resistant tuberculosis, which has become a public health concern in many countries. Where resistance occurs, longer periods of treatment may be required, or more toxic and less powerful medications may have to be used (Mueller and Östergren 2016). So we have both the occurrence of increased costs and a higher likelihood of adverse reactions and ineffective treatment. The particular societal influences on pharmaceutical consumption are illuminatingly illustrated in the case of antibiotics.

Centres for disease control in many countries have developed guidelines to prevent antibiotic resistance, focusing in particular on reducing overall consumption of antibiotics and the appropriate circumstances under which they should be used (Mueller and Östergren 2016). However, despite the endeavours of the World Health Organization (WHO) and national centres of disease control, research has found vast differences in the consumption of antibiotics by country. In 2011, research undertaken in the European Union found that the highest consumption of antibiotics was at the level of just over 42 daily doses per 1000 people in Turkey, and the lowest level of consumption was just over 12 daily doses per 1000 people in the Netherlands. Even countries with shared borders could have dramatic differences: Belgium, bordering the Netherlands, had a consumption of just over 31 daily doses per 1000 people (Mueller and Östergren 2016). A partial explanation for the high level of consumption in Turkey is the ability to purchase antibiotics without a prescription, so people can self-diagnose and self-medicate. But this is not the case in many other countries, so the organisation and culture of health service delivery has an important effect on antibiotic consumption. The specifics of what that is in the case of antibiotic prescribing are not clear, but it is clear that aspects of social organisation have a major impact on how we conduct ourselves in relation to drug consumption. With antibiotics we might expect to have the most standardised and uniform approach to prescribing and consumption, given the great efforts made to obtain compliance to guidelines. Yet the variation in consumption is stark.

## Medications and finance in the Global South and Global North

The case of antibiotic use in the European Union might seem puzzling. For example, we see the relatively wealthy nation-state of the Netherlands having the lowest consumption, whereas we might expect richer countries to have higher consumption. However, higher levels of consumption often suggest inappropriate consumption. The poor having less chance of accessing appropriate medications is more clearly seen in the developing world. The profit motive of drug companies can result in the neglect of diseases of the poor, further exacerbating health inequalities. Attempts to address these inequalities have fostered the development of new institutional forms, such as philanthro-capitalism.

Attempts to address inequalities through pharmaceutical solutions do not always achieve the desired outcome and can disguise deeper social problems.

Diseases suffered by groups marginalised in the global economy, such as tropical diseases like sleeping sickness, Chagas disease and leishmaniasis, tend to be neglected in drug development (De Maio 2014). Tropical diseases have a major impact, leading to around 500,000 deaths a year (De Maio 2014). Their neglect by drug companies indicates inequalities in drug development and consumption, a result of commercial imperatives in drug development. The development of meningitis vaccines in the 1990s illustrates this neglect. In the 1990s, attempts were made by the WHO's department on Immunization, Vaccines and Biologicals to support a vaccine to combat meningitis infections following devastating epidemics in sub-Saharan Africa, mainly caused by meningitis group A (Graham 2016). The vaccine supported was a MenA/C conjugate vaccine for the A and C groups of the disease. However, a rising MenC rate of infection in the United Kingdom (UK) causing a thousand deaths led to resources being diverted to develop a monovalent MenC vaccine. That is, resources were diverted from the poor South to the rich North, where better remuneration for drug development was more likely. During the same period as the UK epidemic, 100,000 people died of meningitis in sub-Saharan Africa (Graham 2016).

The moral discomfort over the neglect of diseases of the Global South has fostered attempts to promote drug research and development that does not solely rely on the pursuit of profit by drug companies. These attempts can, at least on the surface, challenge current models of drug development, which are based on obtaining a profit. The Bill and Melinda Gates Foundation and other philanthropic organisations have contributed to global campaigns against neglected tropical diseases (De Maio 2014). The drug companies GlaxoSmithKline and Merck provide medicines to treat lymphatic filariasis, an infection that causes elephantiasis, for free, with the outcome that millions of children have been saved from infection (De Maio 2014). Whether such outcomes can be sustained long term and whether other diseases receive such charitable solutions from drug companies is to be seen.

The kind of approach taken by what has been called philanthro-capitalists (like the Gates Foundation) to respond to health problems in the Global South often lead to single-disease projects that ignore the social, political and economic determinants of ill health (Graham 2016). Although there may be individual success against specific diseases, this may have little impact on reducing the overall burden of disease in countries with low literacy levels, high rates of malnutrition and lack of clean water and sanitation.

A dilemma made clear from the debates about pharmaceuticals for poor countries and the diseases that have a major impact on them is the clash over intellectual property rights and the sharing of resources to develop new drugs for neglected diseases. It is argued that in order to develop medicines for neglected diseases of the poor, drug companies need incentives to attend to diseases for which market prospects are poor, and to engage in ways that do not tie up intellectual property (Lezaun and Montgomery 2015).

Efforts to provide incentives to drug companies have led to the establishment of a 'plethora of product development partnerships (PDPs)' (Lezaun and Montgomery 2015: 5). PDPs have a goal of linking for-profit and not-for-profit sectors. PDPs are the prioritised organisational form for global health research and development expenditure of the Bill and Melinda Gates Foundation. That Foundation had a profound effect on the development of PDPs when it was established in 2000. PDPs commission drug companies as well as academic institutions in drug discovery research, using resources from state and philanthropic sources (Lezaun and Montgomery 2015). Diverse alliances constitute PDPs, and private goods such as patents and facilities are pooled, rather than being protected by the drug companies.

However, the development of PDPs has not fundamentally changed how drug companies operate. Providing resources and loosening up intellectual property rights in relation to diseases targeting the poor opens up opportunities to gain footholds in countries that also have a middle class, and a middle class with the potential to expand and purchase the products used to treat or prevent non-communicable disease (Lezaun and Montgomery 2015). Connections between drug companies, the state and other corporations are made and brands get established. Philanthro-capital and state funds then support the long-term strategies of drug companies to establish and expand markets; they do not challenge the profit motive and shareholder expectations.

In addition to PDPs, other forms of philanthro-capitalism can shape the delivery of health services in the Global South. Nora Kenworthy provides a detailed analysis of a public-private partnership (PPP) in Lesotho focused on HIV treatment for garment workers, which, when the PPP came to an end, ultimately shifted resources from Lesotho's stretched public health system into the hands of private providers (Kenworthy 2016). In this case, pharmaceutical companies were not directly involved, but pharmaceuticals were identified as the solution, with consequences for workers and the state that I discuss on page 151. I will argue from Kenworthy's interpretation that pharmaceuticals have a power to shape policy in poorer countries, or act as mediators for those wanting to reshape policy.

Lesotho has suffered consistently high HIV prevalence. The garment industry is Lesotho's largest private sector employer, and HIV prevalence is at 40 per cent amongst the largely female workforce in this industry. From the perspective of the garment factories, HIV poses a major productivity problem, with workers missing work to attend clinics and a high workforce turnover due to illness and disease (Kenworthy 2016). Research that was undertaken provided evidence that HIV prevention and treatment services based within factories would benefit workers and the industry, which provided impetus for the creation of factory-based HIV programmes. These programmes could additionally be used to promote the Lesotho garment industry as a site of ethical production, particularly to the United States (US) market. That is, the factories could be portrayed as providing welfare services to workers, and workers who are in particular need of employment.

The PPP consortium consisted of philanthropic funding from the Global Fund to Fight AIDS, Tuberculosis and Malaria and the US brand Gap. Anti-retroviral treatment was provided by Lesotho's government and delivered on-site in factories by private doctors (the rationale for private doctors was to avoid drawing human resources away from Lesotho's public sector). The private doctors and other support services were paid from donations by US corporations and other donor agencies. The immediate outcome for workers was positive, with thousands of workers receiving treatment and care, thus being able to maintain their jobs and take less time off work.

The factories themselves provided space for clinics and salaries for support staff. They supported the initiative as it improved productivity and allowed a premium to be put on their products as they were produced by an HIV-infected workforce, thus appealing to humanitarian consumers in the US. A pharmaceutical solution allowed for marketing strategies to be put in place by major US brands. Kenworthy argues that the focus on HIV treatment 'relieved factories and clothing corporations of a broader responsibility to protect workers' welfare' (Kenworthy 2016), noting in particular the garment industry's reputation for unsafe work practices.

The PPP did not last however, and with its demise factories continued to provide services but deducted doctors' fees from the workers' wages. For most workers this was too costly, and many tried to return to the public health system. However, the public health system could not cope with the thousands of workers seeking help. In her fieldwork, Kenworthy heard stories of workers dying because they could not afford to pay for the factory services. Furthermore, the use of factory doctors fragmented services, with some doctors only focusing on HIV services and no other health services, forcing workers to attend both the factory private system and seek out help for other conditions in the public health system. Private doctors went on to convince the state to fund, at a more rudimentary level, the HIV treatment for workers that the PPP had abandoned, thus establishing a situation in which resources from the public health system were channelled to private doctors.

This case of the garment industry in Lesotho complicates the picture of the profit motive as a driver of pharmaceutical development. In this case, the profit motive is not coming directly from the pharmaceutical industry, but is rather driven by other industrial interests. Philanthropic support became a mediator of channelling resources from a stretched public health system into private hands, with a single disease focus on pharmaceutical treatments being central to this shift of resources. Antiretroviral treatment then became a central means of reshaping health and social systems in Lesotho.

The case of the Lesotho garment industry indicates one attempt by a poorer nation-state trying to balance expensive medications against the dire need for those medications. State solutions to expensive pharmaceuticals in developing countries can take other forms, including opening up competition in an attempt to keep prices down. At an extreme this can lead to the deregulation of the drug market, taking away regulations that limit access to drugs and oversee their quality, as has occurred in Nigeria. Antoine Lentacker notes a curious inversion that takes place when states deregulate the market, whereby drugs that are the most trustworthy in the developed world are likely to be the least trustworthy in the developing world. This is because brand names sell, and are highly sought after on the unregulated market and so are more likely to be the target of counterfeiters or of being sold even if of dubious quality. Thus, the deregulated market in Nigeria has fostered the development of counterfeit drugs, and drugs being sold that are out of date or have been kept in inadequate conditions (Lentacker 2016).

Significant changes have occurred in the financing of drug developments in the Global North as well as in the Global South. Over recent years there have been a number of controversies over sudden increases in the prices of pharmaceuticals. In one case, the drug company Turing Pharmaceuticals, run by an ex-hedge fund manager, acquired a drug used for the treatment of a parasitic infection, Daraprim and increased the price from US$13.50 a tablet to US$750 a tablet (Pollack 2015). Rather than seeing drug price shifts as an outcome of rogue individuals who are insufferably avaricious and callous, it is more insightful to look at the kinds of shifts in the financing of medications.

Danya Glabau (2017) provides a commentary discussing the increase in the price of EpiPens, used to treat serious allergic reactions, from US$100 for the device in 2009 to US$600 in 2016. Glabau argues that this is not explained away as a case of a greedy CEO, but has to be seen in relation to a shareholder revolution in health care in which there has been a shift in ownership of corporations to external shareholders. These shareholders may be banks and investment companies, whose primary goal is raising share prices. One strategy used by pharmaceutical companies to increase the chances of raising share prices is to buy up smaller companies who have promising products or compounds. To purchase these companies, capital is required. Besides having market success with medications, companies can raise capital by raising the stock price, and so improve the financial valuation of the company, providing opportunities to borrow more money. Mylan, the company that produced the EpiPen, used this strategy to acquire MEDA, a Swedish pharmaceutical company. The steep rise in the price of the EpiPen coincided with this strategy, as a part of the valuation of the company was based on anticipated revenue from the EpiPen, the steep rise in price allowed the company to convince investors of a future of increasing returns.

Another strategy to protect profits is to rebrand pharmaceuticals and promote them to treat new disorders, thus protecting the patent. Eli Lilly rebranded Prozac, used for treating depression, as Sarafem, marketing the product as a treatment for premenstrual dysphoric disorder (PMDD). To achieve this outcome the Food and Drug Administration (FDA) had to recognise PMDD as a distinct disease state, which occurred in 1999. With this success Eli Lilly were able to extend the patent of fluoxetine, the main ingredient of both Prozac and the newly branded Sarafem (Ebeling 2011). By protecting its patent, cheaper generic versions of fluoxetine could not come on to the market.

An intriguing connection between the Global North and Global South is made through pharmaceutical buyers' clubs. Mathieu Quet (2018) discusses the development of these clubs that came about in response to drug companies differentially pricing their product in different parts of the world. In 2014, the drug company Gilead was granted approval to market an antiviral therapy against hepatitis C, which consisted of a combination of the drugs Sofosbuvir and Ledipasvir. This combination was claimed to have a cure rate in excess of 80 per cent following a 12-week course. Gilead imposed a price of US$84,000 for a course of this drug in the US. Gilead also signed a licensing agreement with Indian generic manufacturers that allowed the drug combination to be distributed in 90 countries that would cost only US$900 for a course of treatment. The actual cost of manufacture of the drug is estimated at between US$68 and US$136 per course (Quet 2018). In order to avoid 'diversion' of the less expensive drugs from the Global South to the Global North, Gilead requested that the names and phone numbers of patients be recorded, and access to treatment required proof of residence. In addition, each bottle of the drugs had a code that identified the patient. Gilead were not only manufacturing and marketing the drug, but carefully controlling its distribution.

One response to tiered pricing across nation-states has been the development of buyers' clubs. These clubs are organised to import drugs between countries. Generally, buyers' clubs are not profit making organisations, but have been formed in response to a health activism ethic (Quet 2018). Poor people in the Global North and middle income countries could suffer and die from not being able to access expensive drugs that might not be state subsidised. Buyers' clubs are oriented to social justice. Ready communication via the Internet means that buyers' clubs can link up different countries without having to meet in person, and sick individuals do not have to move between countries to collect medications. Medications can be purchased and shipped to those in need.

A clash of logics between the desire to improve the health of populations and prevent premature death and the desire of shareholders to obtain as high a return on investment as is possible is clearly seen in these examples from the Global North. With the dominance of financial capitalism the health of populations is made subordinate to the greater goal of profits and returns for shareholders. In response to concerns about profit gouging and moral turpitude, various solutions have been explored by drug companies and philanthro-capitalists altering the dynamics of capitalism and giving rise to new forms of activism.

## Reaching prescribers and consumers

I have noted that concerns about the quality of pharmaceuticals can be an issue in the Global South, particularly in deregulated drug markets, but quality concerns have become more prominent in the Global North as well, resulting from changing forms of pharmaceutical access. This section outlines some shifts in the strategies used by drug companies to increase the consumption of their products in the Global North, with one consequence being that pharmaceutical users may have quality issues to be concerned about as access to medications is opened up. The shift outlined here is from drug companies targeting doctors, to drug companies targeting patients in order to influence the doctor-patient consultation, to drug companies using cyberpharmacies in ways that can market directly to the patient and exclude doctors altogether. I would like to emphasise that this could perhaps be seen as a return to the marketing strategies of drug companies that occurred in the nineteenth century, where producers of patent medicine, noted in Chapter 2, used the popular press to directly target drug users.

Anthropologist Emily Martin (2006b) interviewed a range of people in the pharmaceutical industry and notes a shift in the focus of drug representatives and drug advertisers over time. In the 1950s and 1960s, executives of the drug company Merck actively sought to educate doctors. For example, in order to get doctors to prescribe their drug Elavil for depression, Merck drug representatives, known as detail men, had to teach doctors to distinguish a diagnosis of anxiety from one of depression. Without such 'education', doctors were more likely to put patients on tranquilisers manufactured by Merck's competitors, rather than on Merck's antidepressant medication. Merck developed a set of target symptoms so that doctors would recognise depression, and doctors did indeed use them, accepting the drug companies as medical educators. In addition to providing this education, Martin found that these old school salespeople and marketers established long-term relationships with these doctors, and focused on advertising in medical journals only accessed by doctors. Forty years later, the focus of drug company sales and marketing was quite different. In an era of direct-to-consumer advertising (DTCA) and direct-to-consumer information (DTCI), the patient now becomes a focus of attention.

Being able to target patients directly allows a change in drug company rhetoric to one that emphasises patient empowerment. In Martin's research, one drug developer argued that half of the people who suffer from migraines are treated with narcotics by doctors, rather than particular migraine drugs that can improve migraines for most sufferers. However, instead of educating doctors on this issue, drug companies now focus on empowering patients directly through the dissemination of marketing materials via the Internet (Martin 2006b). In doing so, the drug companies provide information to patients to take into the consultation in an effort to influence decisions made about the drugs that are prescribed. In Chapter 3, we looked at some of the strategies used on websites to sell pharmaceuticals. In the example discussed, that of Propecia for baldness, tools for self-diagnosis were provided and the stigmatisation of baldness was promoted to influence those accessing the websites to request Propecia from their doctor (Harvey 2013). This is an example of what is termed DTCA.

In 1997, the FDA relaxed rules about DTCA of prescription medicines in the US. New Zealand is the only other country in the world that allows DTCA for prescription medications, although South Korea and Bangladesh have more recently allowed limited DTCA (Ebeling 2011). The FDA places some limits around DTCA. For example, it prohibits, at least in theory, unbalanced presentations where benefits of drugs are prominently displayed whilst risks are hidden away (Biegler and Vargas 2016). The FDA moreover attempts to dictate such issues as the size of print and the information provided on advertisements, which in television advertisements includes regulating the speed and loudness of 'monotone recitations of side effects at the end of the ad' (Martin 2006a: 282). Despite such constraints, drug company spending on DTCA in the US rose from US$1.2 billion per annum to US$5.4 billion from 1998 to 2006. The average US citizen is now exposed to nearly 15 hours of DTCA commercials per year (Biegler and Vargas 2016). Although US citizens still have to obtain prescriptions from medical doctors to access the advertised drugs, research has shown that doctors have a high incidence of assenting to patient drug requests (Biegler and Vargas 2016).

The role of advertisers is to persuade people to purchase a product or more of a product, and the efforts to persuade through DTCA are effective. It has been estimated that DTCA generates US$4 for every US$1 spent. It is unsurprising therefore that there has been such a rapid increase in DTCA spending. However, the goal of selling the product can conflict with the goal of informing people about medications (Biegler and Vargas 2016). Despite the requirements of the FDA to ensure that drug information is balanced, it has no prohibitions around the use of what Paul Biegler and Patrick Vargas (2016) call evaluative conditioning, or what we could simply state as the clever marketing that leads people to believe that medications are more beneficial and more safe than they are.

Biegler and Vargas (2016) suggest that one explanation for the success of DTCA advertising is evaluative conditioning, where favourable attitudes to a product or service is achieved by pairing that product or service with images or sounds that are ordinarily positively received, technically termed images or sounds of positive valence (Biegler and Vargas 2016). Images and music that evoke pleasant feelings not only have a positive emotional effect but can influence people's beliefs. In their experimental study of a fictional drug, Biegler and Vargas found that people who saw the drug paired with positive images were more likely to believe that the drug was safer and more effective than people who saw it paired with neutral or negative images. Positive images used in the research included the use of cute animals and chocolate bars. In addition to DTCA and online pitches to potential patients, drug company promotion work can include disease awareness campaigns, which critics might refer to as disease mongering, the creation and support of advocacy groups that can lobby for the drug companies, and underwriting large sporting events (Ebeling 2011).

Over-the-counter (OTC) drugs are not subject to DTCA regulations and so do not have advertising restrictions placed on them. A number of countries have made significant shifts in changing the status of many drugs from prescription only to OTC, including the UK (Abraham 2009) and France (Fainzang 2017). Such moves may be undertaken using a rhetoric of patient empowerment, but OTC medications can be driven by the attempts by states to reduce expenditure on drugs as they incur out-of-pocket payments from consumers and so reduce state costs.

In addition to the rise of DTCA in the US and New Zealand and some of the potential problems it raises in changing the dynamics of the doctor-patient relationship that was noted in the case study of Propecia, there has been the appearance of cyberpharmacies that further change this relationship. Cyberpharmacies promote the shift from drug users as patients to drug users as customers. Cyberpharmacies, which started appearing in the late 1990s, are websites through which customers can purchase medicines, including prescription medicine (Orizio and Gelatti 2010). Cyberpharmacies use a number of arguments to convince people to purchase their products, including the ability to avoid doctors, drugs being cheaper, the possibility of trying out different drugs to see what works for them and the ability to purchase anonymously. The latter is likely to be important for issues that might attract embarrassment, such as erectile dysfunction (Orizio and Gelatti 2010) or sexually transmitted diseases (Fainzang 2017).

Cyberpharmacies have been regarded by the WHO and national public health organisations as a serious public health threat (Orizio and Gelatti 2010). In many jurisdictions it is legal to purchase prescription medications online with a prescription, but some cyberpharmacies provide drugs without prescriptions, and there are many drugs available that do not require prescriptions. Concerns over access to prescription medications without a prescription have led to attempts by national and supranational agencies, like the European Union, to prohibit such purchases online (Orizio and Gelatti 2010). However, it is difficult to police such a prohibition. The availability of online purchasing of drugs can take pharmacists and medical doctors out of the loop, changing the nature of pharmaceuticalised governance as anonymous online shopping entrepreneurs come into the relationship with drug users.

Online purchasing raises concerns about self-medication that might not be in the patient's best interests. Studies have been undertaken where researchers place orders for prescription medicines through these pharmacies and their purchases have been honoured. In some of this research, the researchers filled out online questionnaires, providing information that would be a contraindication for the prescription of the drug, but the researchers were still able to purchase it (Orizio and Gelatti 2010). Additional concerns have been raised over the appropriate storage of cyberpharmacy stock and safe transportation, in addition to concerns about counterfeit drugs (Orizio and Gelatti 2010). Customs seizures of pharmaceuticals in the US found that two-thirds of drugs purchased overseas by patients were either not approved by the FDA or had been taken off the market, and that 5 per cent had no active ingredient (Rajagopal 2016).

The debates around cyberpharmacies can be considered dilemmatic. On one hand, cyberpharmacies facilitate patient empowerment and choice and freedom from medical domination; on the other, they empower pharmaceutical companies and facilitate self-prescribing and its associated dangers. There are reasons why some drugs are prescription only, including avoiding unnecessary drug consumption, and having expert medical oversight in determining the balance of benefits and harms from drugs (Orizio and Gelatti 2010). The

presence of cyberpharmacies supports the view that there has been a funda-
mental shift in our relationship to health care, where patients have been transformed to customers. This argument is often made with a neo-Foucauldian
framing that, we are neoliberal subjects who have been made responsible for our
own health care choices and medical practice, and health care activities have
become more market-driven (Gabe *et al.* 2015).

Arguably the shift in the Global North to patients as customers has some parallels with the de-regulation of drug markets in some parts of the Global South.
Both developments fit broadly within what has been called neoliberalism, with
the freeing up of markets and the valorisation of consumer choice (Gabe *et al.*
2015). The drivers for freeing up markets may come from different sources
though: developments in the Global North are shaped by drug companies
expanding their market, whilst in the Global South they are shaped by states
attempting to rein in the costs of health care.

## Citizens and pharmaceuticals

Pharmaceutical companies have an obvious investment in obtaining the best possible image for their medications, and so the presentation of how these medications may transform our lives is a common strategy, seen in various examples
throughout this book including the example of Propecia medication in Chapter 3
and claims made in DTCA noted on page 155. Sociological analyses can be critical of such representations, but sociologists have also been concerned with the
transformative impact of pharmaceuticals on identity and behaviours of users.

Asha Persson (2016) utilises the concept of pharmaceutical citizenship in her
research on the re-imagining of HIV in a time of treatment-as-prevention. Pharmaceutical citizenship alludes to the idea that pharmacological treatment can be
pivotal to citizenship that is, to a person being able to engage actively in society.
In the case of HIV, trials have shown a near 100 per cent reduction in the sexual
transmission of the infection in heterosexual serodiscordant couples (where one
partner is HIV-positive and the other is not) as a result of effective antiretroviral
treatment. Antiretroviral treatment thus, has the potential to reconfigure HIV
from being one of the most contagious infections to one that is harmless; from a
public health perspective, advocating for adherence to antiretroviral treatment
becomes a major plank in eliminating the infection. At an interpersonal level,
issues of trust change for serodiscordant couples. For the uninfected partner,
unprotected sex could now be a reasonable risk as long as the infected partner
could be trusted to take the medications (Persson 2016). Safe sex is transformed
as medication is the focus of prophylaxis, as opposed to the use of condoms. The
stigma of HIV infection is lessened as aspects of sexual belonging are restored
(Persson 2016).

Persson undertook her research in Australia. The scenario can be very
different in less wealthy countries. Cousins' ethnographic research in South
Africa found that for some people, taking antiretroviral treatment could itself
have life-threatening consequences. In Cousins' study, HIV-positive South

Africans were eligible for a disability grant, but only if their CD4 count – a measure of immune system functioning – was below 200. If treatment meant their CD4 count rose above 200 they would lose that grant, and for some losing that grant meant no longer having the resources to purchase food. A nutritionally adequate diet would have to be sacrificed if HIV treatment was to be maintained (Cousins 2016).

Persson's and Cousins' ethnographies provide dramatic contrasts in pharmaceutical relations. The faces of pharmaceutical governance are not alike. The pharmaceutical intervention of antiretroviral treatment may transform behaviours and relationships in positive ways in the Global North, and may exacerbate the marginalised existence for some in the Global South.

## Concluding comments

In this chapter, I have considered a number of different ways in which social organisation shapes drug development, but in addition noting how drug development shapes people and states. Pharmaceutical companies and the drugs they produce shape relationships between people and states in important ways. How these relationships play out can differ dramatically, and in this chapter some differences between the Global North and the Global South illustrate these contrasts.

How pharmaceuticalised governance manifests cannot be divorced from the structures in which drugs are embedded. The production, reproduction and exacerbation of social inequalities worldwide influence what pharmaceuticals are developed and how they are developed. Policy decisions about drug availability intersect with other forms of welfare provision. Decisions about when and how to use pharmaceuticals by citizens, and how those decisions might change relationships with other people and other institutions, are particular to the social formations in which those decisions are made. What might work in positive ways in the Global North, for example, may have negative consequences in the Global South.

Pharmaceuticals can play a crucial role in promoting particular forms of political governance, as with the shift of resources form the public to the private sector in Lesotho. Social policy is shaped in specific ways when pharmaceuticals are viewed as a solution to social problems. But even with different policy drivers we might, at times, see similar outcomes for citizens, as with the potential exposure to low quality or counterfeit drugs in both the Global North and the Global South.

This chapter alerts us to some of the variability in pharmaceuticalised governance, and I have noted the importance of the particular forms of social organisation and nation-state circumstances in explaining variability. The following chapter too considers variability in pharmaceuticalised governance, but shifts the focus to the spaces and sites of resistance to pharmaceuticalisation.

# References

Abraham, J. (2009). Partial progress: Governing the pharmaceutical industry and the NHS, 1948–2008. *Journal of Health Politics Policy and Law* 34: 931–977.

Biegler, P. and Vargas, P. (2016). Feeling is believing: Evaluative conditioning and the ethics of pharmaceutical advertising. *Bioethical Inquiry* 13: 271–279.

Brown, B. and Crawford, P. (2009). 'Post antibiotic apocalypse': Discourses of mutation in narratives of MRSA. *Sociology of Health and Illness* 31: 508–524.

Cousins, T. (2016). Antiretroviral therapy and nutrition in Southern Africa: Citizenship and the grammar of hunger. *Medical Anthropology* 35: 433–446.

De Maio F. (2014). *Global Health Inequities: A Sociological Perspective.* Basingstoke: Palgrave Macmillan.

Ebeling, M. (2011). 'Get with the program!': Pharmaceutical marketing, symptom check-lists and self-diagnosis. *Social Science and Medicine* 73: 825–832.

Fainzang, S. (2017). *Self-Medication and Society: Mirages of Autonomy.* Abingdon: Routledge.

Gabe, J., Harley, K. and Calnan, M. (2015). Healthcare choice: Discourses, perceptions, experiences and practices. *Current Sociology* 63: 623–635.

Glabau, D. (2017). Conflicting assumptions: The meaning of price in the pharmaceutical economy. *Science as Culture* 26: 455–467.

Graham, J. (2016). Ambiguous capture: Collaborative capitalism and the Meningitis Vaccine Project. *Medical Anthropology* 35: 419–432.

Harvey, K. (2013). Medicalisation, pharmaceutical promotion and the Internet: A critical multimodal discourse analysis of hair loss websites. *Social Semiotics* 23: 691–714.

Kenworthy, N. (2016). Governing through production: A public-private partnership's impacts and dissolution in Lesotho's garment industry. In: *Case Studies on Corporations and Global Health Governance: Impacts, Influences and Accountability* (eds N. Kenworthy, R. MacKenzie and K. Lee), 11–25. London: Rowman and Littlefield.

Lentacker, A. (2016). The symbolic economy of drugs. *Social Studies of Science* 46: 140–156.

Lezaun, J. and Montgomery, C. (2015). The pharmaceutical commons: Sharing and exclusion in global health drug development. *Science, Technology and Human Values* 40: 3–29.

Martin, E. (2006a). The pharmaceutical person. *BioSocieties* 1: 273–287.

Martin, E. (2006b). Pharmaceutical virtue. *Culture, Medicine and Psychiatry* 30: 157–174.

Mueller, T. and Östergren, P-O. (2016). The correlation between regulatory conditions and antibiotic consumption within the WHO European Region. *Health Policy* 120: 882–889.

Orizio, G. and Gelatti, U. (2010). Public eHealth and new scenarios in terms of risks and opportunities: A specific focus on cyberpharmacies. *Social Semiotics* 2: 29–41.

Persson, A. (2016). 'The world has changed': Pharmaceutical citizenship and the reimagining of serodiscordant sexuality among couples with mixed HIV status in Australia. *Sociology of Health and Illness* 38: 380–395.

Pollack, A. (2015). Drug goes from $13.50 a tablet to $750, overnight. *New York Times* (20 September).

Quet, M. (2018). Pharmaceutical capitalism and its logistics: Access to hepatitis C treatment. *Theory, Culture and Society* 35: 67–89.

Rajagopal, M. (2016). Internet pharmacies – boon or threat? *Progress in Neurology and Psychiatry* 20 (5): 4–5. http://onlinelibrary.wiley.com/doi/10.1002/pnp.1438/pdf.

# 12 Resisting pharmaceuticalised governance

Some of the research observations noted in Chapters 4 and 5 suggest that, although many people see drugs as restorative and even as integrated into their personal physiologies, many others resist medications on a number of grounds. The observation that people do resist medications has been noted in other research. Those who resist pharmaceuticals have been categorised as rejectors (Dowell and Hudson 1997; Pound *et al.* 2005). Some users actively modify their prescribed pharmaceutical regimes, as Pandora Pound and colleagues note (Pound *et al.* 2005) and as I noted in Chapter 5. Many participants in our research claimed to avoid medications when they could. Tony stated that he 'won't take pills' and Paul would try 'just any other alternative rather than taking drugs' (Chamberlain *et al.* 2011: 301). Medications might be resisted because of their side effects, or their potential to cause unwanted long-term effects on the body, or they might be resisted because they do not deal with what people believe to be the 'true cause' of the problem (Chamberlain *et al.* 2011: 304). Some participants in our research, discussed in Chapters 4 to 6, took a cynical attitude to pharmaceutical advertising, for example, describing a weight loss advertisement as 'total quackery'. They were cynical of the attempts of drug companies to provide false hope and position potential purchasers of drugs as having some deficit with claims that 'if you do this then your life will be better' (Hodgetts *et al.* 2017: 3554). This cynicism is an expression of agency by householders.

In this chapter, I consider a variety of forms of resistance. I start by considering the possibilities for de-pharmaceuticalisation and I suggest that it is unlikely that, at a societal level we will see much evidence of de-pharmaceuticalisation. However, this does not mean that resistance to pharmaceuticalised governance does not occur within society, as has been noted with householders resisting and modifying pharmaceutical use. The example of psychotropic drugs is used to explore a variety of ways in which people resist being pharmaceuticalised and some of the reasons for that resistance, including the shame of diagnosis and challenges to diagnosis. Cancer treatment, often used in the face of potentially terminal illness, provides us with different examples of how pharmaceuticalised governance is resisted, with reactions against the toxicity of drugs and the seeking out of alternative approaches to treatment. I follow this by considering how resistance can occur at an institutional level, with drug regulatory agencies playing an ambiguous role that plays out in a variety of ways. Finally, I consider resistance at an ideological level through the example of alternative therapies, focusing on the case of homeopathy to illustrate contrasting understandings of disease and treatment to that of orthodox pharmaceutical approaches.

I suggest that resistance to pharmaceuticals is commonplace, but its impact is limited. Processes of medicalisation and pharmaceuticalisation appear to be on an inexorable trajectory.

## De-medicalisation and de-pharmaceuticalisation

The view that our lives are becoming increasingly medicalised and pharmaceuticalised is a compelling one. There are, however, historical examples where we can see the reversal of this trend. Some diagnostic categories go out of favour, and without a diagnosis a behaviour, activity or condition can be de-medicalised. De-medicalisation, though not necessarily de-pharmaceuticalisation, is seen in the rise and fall of the diagnosis of masturbatory insanity. From our perspective in the twenty-first century we might assume that the idea that masturbation could lead to mental disorder was only held by a few marginal physicians and that it was not widely regarded as a credible hypothesis, but in Britain and the United States (US) in the eighteenth and nineteenth centuries masturbation was regarded as a frequent cause of mental illness (Hare 1962). Edward Hare, psychiatrist and historian, provided a detailed account of the hold that the masturbation hypothesis had on the medical profession.

The chronic masturbator was thought to go into a state of fatigue, following which a number of disorders could develop such as melancholy, dementia, catalepsy and imbecility. This hypothesis started to be contested by the later 1800s but still appeared in textbooks in the 1930s. The treatments for masturbatory insanity were not the most successful. After initial attempts at moral exhortation and dietary and activity changes, other chemical, surgical and mechanical options were tried over time. Bromide of potassium was tried. With a lack of success women might suffer clitoridectomy. Men might have their prepuce blistered or silver rings used to prevent retraction of the prepuce. Some were even castrated as a form of treatment.

The reason for the decline in the credibility of this hypothesis can be speculated upon, but was facilitated by surveys of the population that found that masturbation was much more widely practised than had been thought, so the idea that it caused insanity could not be generally accepted. I would add to this speculation and suggest that the lack of a pharmaceutical treatment for the 'disease' took one important player out of the picture, the drug companies that could have profited by curing the population of masturbation.

Another example of de-medicalisation is homosexuality. Many health professionals viewed homosexuality as a pathological condition requiring therapeutic intervention. It was a category of disease listed in the *Diagnostic and Statistical Manual of Mental Disorders: DSM-II* (American Psychiatric Association 1968). After a process of intense lobbying this categorisation was removed in 1980.

De-medicalisation, therefore can occur where something once regarded as being in the medical domain is no longer seen as part of that domain, but I am not aware of it occurring in a situation of successful pharmaceuticalisation. What I mean by successful is a situation where a pharmaceutical has been regarded by health professionals and patients as having a positive effect on a diagnosed condition. That is, I suggest that where a drug is used in treatment, de-medicalisation seems less likely. De-medicalisation occurs, but it is more difficult to find examples of de-pharmaceuticalisation. The most obvious examples of de-medicalisation, as noted here, relate to the initial medicalisation of activities that attracted moral opprobrium, and with changes in morals and values in societies a process of de-medicalisation becomes possible. In situations where pharmaceuticalisation has occurred the interests of drug companies, health practitioners and others coalesce to maintain an understanding that pharmaceuticals are the solution. As was discussed in Chapter 3, a common path is then to expand the population base targeted by the pharmaceutical solution.

We are unlikely to see a broad trend of de-pharmaceuticalisation in society, but nevertheless there are some examples of it happening at an individual level. The accounts of household use of pharmaceuticals discussed in Chapters 4 to 6 provide many examples of individual householders resisting advice from health professionals and not consuming medications as advised. Sylvie Fainzang, in her study of self-medication practices by people in Paris, France, observes processes of interpretation and diagnosis from lay people, and documents individual acts of de-medicalisation, with for example, someone not following medical advice to take antibiotics and instead changing her diet in response to a throat problem (Fainzang 2017). Support groups may grow up around rejections of the pharmaceuticalisation of certain conditions. In response to the pharmaceuticalisation of shyness through the establishment of social anxiety disorder as a category of disease, websites and support groups advocating for introverts and those who enjoy quiet and solitude have arisen (Collin 2016). The ways in which people can form collectives around diagnostic labels, medication use or in this case resistance to diagnostic labels, has variously been referred to as biosociality and bio-citizenship (Collin 2016).

## Psychological therapies and resistance to psychotropic drugs

Responses to psychotropic and neuroleptic drugs provide a window to different forms of resistance to pharmaceuticals, which can occur at both an individual and ideological level. In general, resistance to long-term pharmaceutical treatments has been deemed a worldwide problem (Britten *et al.* 2010). In relation to psychotropic drugs, non-adherence can be viewed by health professionals as a symptom of mental illness and as a reason for involuntary hospitalisation. In a review of resistance to psychotropic medications, Nicky Britten and colleagues note a range of reasons for resistance, including the stigma of the condition (particularly the case with a diagnosis of schizophrenia) and the stigma of taking medications, different understandings of the cause of mental illness (e.g. as an outcome of particular personal circumstances that need to be changed, rather than use medication), a desire to avoid embarrassing side effects like weight gain or tremors, and a desire to resist social control. Some users desired normality and felt they could not feel normal if they had to rely on pharmaceuticals. As with our research on medications in the household, Britten and colleagues suggest that, from the evidence of the research they looked at, non-adherence to psychotropic drugs was often a purposeful action, and resulting from considerable effort on the part of users to evaluate the effects of drugs and their non-use (Britten *et al.* 2010).

In Chapter 8, I noted that people suffering from some mental distress may be fearful of consulting a health professional. One reason can be concerns about the effects that treatment might have on them. Fainzang finds similar concerns in some of her participants who self-medicate, including avoiding doctors for 'fear of getting caught in a cycle of medical care and a regular and onerous prescription of psychoactive drugs' (Fainzang 2017: 57). In our research on households, there were examples where people made clear distinctions between psychotropic drugs and other medications. Melanie did not always adhere to her psychotropic medication regime because she felt that these particular drugs were 'poisoning my body', but she did not have similar problems with medications for her heart and for diabetes (Chamberlain *et al.* 2011: 304).

People who do go on to take psychotropic drugs can be in two minds about them. We noted in Chapter 4 the relationships to psychotropic drugs that Kim and Sophie had. For Sophie, one had to take responsibility in relation to the drugs. Kim would get to the point of rebellion against taking the drugs because they affected such things as her levels of energy and weight. In Emily Martin's study, focusing on psychotropic drugs, she argues that people's accounts of using these drugs are deeply ambivalent. People feel both repulsed and attracted to them, and where some symptoms are eased but new ones might appear (Martin 2006).

Lisa Blackman (2012) notes another form of resistance to drugs from many people who hear voices. Blackman's mother had the experience of hearing voices, and attempts by medical professionals to suppress these voices included the use of drugs and electroconvulsive therapy. The hearing of voices is usually a central component in a diagnosis of schizophrenia. The voices themselves are conventionally seen as some kind of sensory phenomena related to a malfunction in the brain, occurring when the capacity to self-monitor one's inner speech is defective. From this perspective, the voices themselves and what they said was meaningless. This kind of interpretation was seriously challenged in the 1980s and 1990s with the work of two Dutch psychiatrists, Marius Romme and Sandra Escher. Romme and Escher were involved early on in the establishment of The Hearing Voices Network, which took voices seriously, as in, believing that they should be listened to (Blackman 2012). This idea challenges contemporary psychiatric understandings and pharmaceutical practices, but it can additionally challenge our perceptions of the body and mind.

Blackman suggests that there are different ways of considering hallucinatory phenomena, such as understanding voices as an outcome of the suppression of trauma or of intergenerational transmission of trauma. She draws on the experiences of Korean women who became the brides of US military personnel as an example of this, arguing that their hearing of voices and experience of psychosis can be interpreted as a manifestation of the trauma from their profound shame that was never discussed or talked about. These traumatic secrets can go on to haunt the next generation. Blackman develops the argument that instead of perception being bound to a single, closed psychological subject, perception can be distributed collectively. This kind of thinking would seem to undermine the idea that treatment should focus on an individual in order to control their symptoms or perceptual problems. The Hearing Voices Network can help people respond to this sense that they are not a single-bounded unitary subject, but are both one and many (Blackman 2012).

## Resistance in the face of terminal illness

Cancer is a disease that, when diagnosed, is likely to evoke fear and dread. It is, furthermore, a site of extremes of treatment. For many cancers, a conventional medical approach is chemotherapy, the use of highly toxic drugs to try to eliminate any traces of cancer. Other treatments can be equally as taxing, such as radiotherapy and surgery. It can only be expected that in the face of such toxic and at times debilitating treatments that have variable success rates, many would turn to alternative approaches and resist pharmaceuticalisation.

Resistance of this type can lead to extraordinary stand-offs between patients or their families and medical professionals. An example of this is the Liam Williams-Holloway case that occurred in New Zealand during 1999 and 2000. In this case, medical practitioners were pitted against a family over the treatment of a child with cancer. The family went into hiding so that they could provide alternative treatment for their child, and the medical oncologists took legal action to make Liam a ward of court so that he could be compelled to receive orthodox treatment (Broom 2000). This case polarised public opinion on the use of alternative therapies for cancer, with some suggesting that it is a family's right to seek out the treatment they believe is best for their child, and others suggesting that designated experts should decide what is best.

As will be discussed on page 173, it is common for people to use both alternative approaches and conventional approaches to treat conditions, and this is also the case with cancer. It has been estimated that between 20 and 60 per cent of cancer patients use complementary and alternative medicines (CAM) (Broom and Tovey 2008). The use of CAM in the face of cancer has been seen to have positive aspects, such as providing a sense of empowerment and control for patients and promoting hope. Many people combine chemotherapy and other aggressive medical approaches with meditation practices, mindfulness and mental imaging, and these practices have been associated with longer than expected survival (Cunningham *et al.* 2000). Research on exceptional cancer survivors found that in addition to conventional approaches, patients used a variety of CAM approaches, which Johanna Hök and colleagues (2009) classified as energy-based therapies, biologically-based therapies, manipulative therapies and body-based therapies. Hök and colleagues found that both biomedical health practitioners and alternative healing practitioners attributed patient survival with cancer to their own interventions, however, the patients who saw both, attributed survival to combinations of conventional and alternative treatments and their own actions and decisions, or agency.

In this book, I have focused on how the use of pharmaceuticals in everyday life brings into play different forms of self-governance, or pharmaceuticalised governance. Many dimensions of this have been explored, and the particular ways in which this plays out at broad cultural, institutional and interactional levels. But any therapeutic regime requires forms of self-governance, although they are likely to take different shapes from that of pharmaceutical governance as there are different social forces at play. Using CAM brings into play particular forms of self-governance. Cancer survival strategies for those post-diagnosis are entwined with imperatives to diet and exercise to prevent recurrence and progression of disease (Bell 2010). Some negative effects of such imperatives are illustrated by Alex Broom and Philip Tovey in their discussion of the use of CAM in cases of incurable cancer (Broom and Tovey 2008). In some situations, the use of alternative approaches can be at great personal and financial cost. They highlight one case of a man in his 80s who undertakes a very rigorous and costly dietary regime and the use of enemas to detoxify his body in an unsuccessful effort to keep the cancer at bay. The demands to take responsibility, and in this case to put so much energy into what was a futile attempt to extend life, takes its toll on individuals and their families.

Tensions can develop when there are clashes between cancer health professionals and patients over the use of non-biomedical approaches. An example of this is noted in Chapter 6, where a clash between a Māori cancer patient and her oncologist over her desire to use a traditional Māori approach to therapeutics was discussed. In that instance, the patient had been to a Māori healer who said she would help her, but that her condition looked like cancer so she should have it checked out by her 'Pākehā [non-Māori] doctor'. The patient 'didn't trust the western medical system' because in her view it belittled Māori medicine, and people were still dying under western medical treatment. When she mentioned her desire to pursue an unconventional approach to cancer treatment, her oncologist was not supportive, and this led to her walking out of the consultation. She stated in relation to orthodox medical approaches that:

> Māori patients who've gone that way have died, and I tried to tell him a lot of Pākehā patients that have gone that way have died too ... in fact I thought more people have died under the knife than under the holistic approach. So I just thought he had the cheek ... it has never left my memory.

Here we have a situation where relationships between the patient and her health professional have broken down because of a sense that the patient's approach is being belittled. The patient's resistance could of course have major consequences for her. But in this research we also saw other situations, for example, where in a case that seemed particularly difficult, the cancer health professional was quite happy for the patient to pursue an alternative approach (Dew *et al.* Forthcoming).

Moana (a pseudonym) is attending a radiation oncology consultation. She has chronic obstructive pulmonary disease and severely reduced activities. Any treatment related to a likely lung tumour is unlikely to be helpful, and may cause further damage to the lungs. But Moana has to make a decision about whether to go with some treatment that might have a small chance of helping or give up on treatment altogether. Moana makes a decision (quite rare in cancer care consultations, where many 'decisions' are more like informing patients of a treatment plan) to try out an alternative approach: 'apricot kernels, seeds … vitamins and all that sort of thing'. She states that by the next appointment 'I will have done a course of it, and we'll see where we are'. The oncologist does not challenge this decision, even though from a conventional perspective it would be seen as a waste of time and effort. The oncologist allows this course of action in the face of having nothing of substance to offer himself (Dew *et al.* Forthcoming). In this instance, de-medicalisation occurs at a patient level as a result of a lack of any pharmaceutical or medical solution.

## State resistance

Occasionally the funding of cancer drugs is a prominent public issue. Cancer patient lobby groups may advocate for further pharmaceuticalisation of cancer treatment, and governments may resist pharmaceuticalisation if it means paying out for expensive new medications. The research team I worked with that provided the material for discussions in Chapters 4 and 5 looked at the controversy around a drug with the brand name of Herceptin (Gabe *et al.* 2012). Herceptin is a drug used in the treatment of early stage breast cancer. The agency responsible for managing the list of prescription pharmaceutical products that are subsidised by the state in the New Zealand health care system, called PHARMAC, had determined in 2006 that Herceptin could be subsidised for a nine-week period. They took this stance on the basis of the evidence available to them that the longer course of treatment provided no extra benefits and there were concerns about the cardiotoxicity of the drug.

Herceptin costs NZ$50,000 per year per patient. The difference in cost between a nine-week course and a 12-month course is therefore quite substantial. Roche, who manufactured Herceptin, were not happy with PHARMAC's refusal to fund 12-month courses. Roche challenged PHARMAC's cost-benefit analysis in a letter to the *New Zealand Medical Journal* and made submissions to the High Court during a judicial review of PHARMAC decision-making (Gabe *et al.* 2012). Roche's endeavours were supported by some scientists and medical researchers and by a lobby group advocating for women with breast cancer. Although there is no evidence that Roche was involved in the lobby group, in the United Kingdom (UK) the company had contacted women with breast cancer to ask them to help to get the drug funded (Abraham 2009).

A number of women with HER2 positive breast cancer took PHARMAC to court in an attempt to get PHARMAC to fund Herceptin for the 12-month course. The High Court noted concerns about the consultation process used by PHARMAC and ordered PHARMAC to undertake another consultation process and then review its decision. PHARMAC complied but came to the same conclusion, providing a point of resistance to further pharmaceuticalisation.

Media attention focused on those women who wanted the 12-month course and who would have to somehow raise the tens of thousands of dollars required to pay for it. The power of such presentations of women with a deadly disease in desperate circumstances was used by one of the major political parties, with the National Party, a pro-business party, promising to fund Herceptin for 12 months if elected. After being elected in 2008, this promise was kept. As PHARMAC refused to play ball, the funding of the drug was made available through a different agency, the Ministry of Health. The annual cost of funding Herceptin in New Zealand, a country of 4.5 million people, came in at just under NZ$40 million annually (Brown 2017).

Research into the best length of time to take Herceptin to provide optimal results and minimise adverse reactions was ongoing. In 2017, it was reported that a trial of over 2000 women across seven countries concluded that the nine-week course was as effective as the 12-month course, with the shorter course having fewer side effects, being less inconvenient and costing less (Brown 2017). In the meantime, the New Zealand government had filled Roche's coffers with many millions of dollars.

## Muted institutional resistance

The case of PHARMAC resisting pressure to fund Herceptin illustrates the possibilities of resistance to expanded pharmaceuticalisation from those agencies responsible for appraising the effectiveness of drugs and making recommendations on their use. In England and Wales, this role is undertaken by the National Institute for Health and Care Excellence (NICE). The consequence of NICE drug recommendations is that the drugs must be made available by National Health Service Trusts (Brown and Calnan 2010). NICE could resist making recommendations for drugs of marginal benefit. As noted in Chapter 8, this opportunity is by no means always taken, with David Healy arguing that NICE ignored evidence about the adverse effects of some antipsychotic drugs (Healy 2006). Abraham suggests that government drug regulatory agencies in the UK are biased in favour of the drug companies (Abraham 2009).

In 1949, prior to the establishment of NICE, a Joint Committee on Prescribing was established by the British Ministry of Health to try to restrict the prescribing of medicines that were overly expensive or of little value (Abraham 2009). In 1964, a Committee on the Safety of Drugs was established to advise manufacturers and the government about drug safety but the Committee had no legal powers. It relied on cooperation from the pharmaceutical industry in relation to any recommendations and in fostering relationships with the industry the

Committee treated their deliberations as confidential and undertook rapid reviews to facilitate getting drugs quickly to market (Abraham 2009). John Abraham refers to these concerns by regulatory agencies for the interests of the industry as corporate bias (Abraham 2009). Abraham argues that corporate bias is evident in the regulation of drug safety over time in the UK, noting, for example, that it was not until 2006 that members of such regulatory committees were prohibited from having financial interests in pharmaceutical firms. The close historical relationships between the regulatory bodies in the UK and the drug companies may explain the fact that, between 1972 and 1991, twice as many prescription drugs had to be withdrawn from the UK market as from the US market (Abraham 2009). In essence, the resistance provided by UK drug regulatory agencies to the pharmaceutical industry has been muted to say the least.

The escalating consumption of drugs and the high price of newly introduced pharmaceuticals have provided some greater impetus to rein in drug use. The UK has, since 1957, had a Pharmaceutical Price Regulation Scheme (PPRS). The Scheme has two conflicting objectives: to secure the provision of safe and effective medicines, and to promote a profitable pharmaceutical industry so that drug research and development can be sustained (Abraham 2009). To ensure the latter, drug company profit targets are negotiated between the PPRS and the drug companies, but there is a wide leeway if companies go over this target and make more profit than was agreed. The UK system of pricing has wide implications, with many other countries setting their prices in reference to the UK system (Abraham 2009).

Abraham illustrates the corporate bias that exists in his discussion of a drug marketed for the treatment of influenza. In 1999, NICE recommended that the drug, Relenza, should not be used as it was likely to have very little effect. The manufacturer, Glaxo Wellcome and other drug companies subsequently threatened to shift their laboratories away from the UK. Subsequently NICE changed its position to recommend the drug for use in at-risk individuals (Abraham 2009).

Those making appraisals and guidelines are not, however, simple dupes of the industry, and may provide a source of resistance to pharmaceutical company efforts to persuade committee members. Michael Calnan and colleagues (Calnan *et al.* 2017) undertook an ethnographic study of NICE appraisals of new expensive drugs. They note a number of sources of uncertainty for those involved in the appraisal about the evidence provided by the drug companies in the appraisal process. Uncertainty may result from scepticism about the randomised controlled trial process along the lines I discussed in Chapter 8, and suspicion of the motives of drug company representatives. Appraisers might question how trustworthy the evidence was. They can therefore, provide some resistance to the claims being made by drug companies. That is, within the institutional arrangements for drug appraisal in the UK, resistance to pharmaceuticals could occur. However, taking into account Abraham's claims about corporate bias, any resistance sits within a system designed to support the pharmaceutical companies.

## Resisting corporate bias

The situation in New Zealand is quite different, where the presence of the pharmaceutical industry on the ground is small, and where resistance to pharmaceuticals is established at an institutional level, even if still in a somewhat muted way. In the New Zealand context, PHARMAC mentioned on page 166, can be seen as having a contradictory role in relation to pharmaceuticalisation of the population, but unlike the UK system it is not required to ensure drug company profitability. PHARMAC both promotes the consumption of drugs and resists the expansion of pharmaceutical markets. PHARMAC's brief is to promote the optimal use of medicines. Recommendations about what is optimal may mean actually reducing pharmaceutical consumption in some situations. To do this it determines what medicines attract a state subsidy on the basis of what medicines are likely to give most benefit and at the best price. To enhance cost-effectiveness, PHARMAC enters into negotiation with pharmaceutical companies.

PHARMAC tempers profit gouging by drug companies through a number of different means, for example, using the threat of loss of market share to force product suppliers to compete on price (Zhong 2003). PHARMAC achieves this by grouping together drugs that it deems to produce similar effects in treating a condition, and tends to list on the Pharmaceutical Schedule only one drug in the group to be subsidised. Unsubsidised drugs can still be available to patients, but consumers of the drug have to pay a surcharge, which means those drugs gain very little market share. Drug companies are thus, thrown into competition to provide the lowest price to PHARMAC so that their drug is the one to get on to the Pharmaceutical Schedule.

New drugs are usually only subsidised by PHARMAC if they offer a price lower than the currently subsidised drug. This is a very intensive form of what is called reference pricing. Other countries use reference pricing, but in a different way. Some European systems of reference pricing are based on the average cost of the drug in the therapeutic group. That is, the reference price is an average price. But PHARMAC determines reference pricing on the basis of the lowest cost at which drug companies are willing to supply their drug (Woodfield 2001). So in order to obtain a subsidy a new drug has to be cheaper than the one drug that PHARMAC subsidises. In the US, drug pricing control is in the hands of the drug companies themselves (Martin 2006). PHARMAC uses other strategies as well, such as fixed expenditure caps and tendering for supply, but the detail of these other strategies are not required to make the point clear: a government drug buying agency can, paradoxically, be a source of resistance to some aspects of pharmaceuticalisation, in particular, a lower expenditure on drugs occurs in New Zealand because of its strong regulatory system (Dew and Davis 2014). To illustrate, between 2002 and 2012 PHARMAC assessed that it had achieved savings of NZ\$3.8 billion (Neuwelt *et al.* 2015).

PHARMAC's tactics are not well received by drug companies, and we see criticisms of PHARMAC along similar lines to the attacks on the use of clinical trials overseen by the Food and Drug Administration discussed in Chapter 2.

For example, drug companies complain that if other countries adopted New Zealand's approach there would not be enough resources to develop new drugs (Moore *et al.* 1996). Merck Sharp & Dohme believed the price negotiated for its cholesterol-lowering drug, simvastatin, had reached such a low level in New Zealand that it changed its brand name from Zocor to Lipex because there was a perceived risk of less regulated countries importing the sought after brand name drug at cheaper prices from New Zealand (Begg *et al.* 2003).

The potential for a free trade agreement between New Zealand and the US provoked debate over the continuation of PHARMAC's role as a monopoly purchaser of state subsidised pharmaceuticals in New Zealand. The release of confidential American Embassy diplomatic cables by WikiLeaks in late 2010 illustrated frustration from international pharmaceutical companies with New Zealand's pharmaceutical management (The New Zealand Herald 2010). In free trade agreement negotiating documents, the US sought to undermine reference pricing and increase the role of the drug industry in drug regulation decision-making (Neuwelt *et al.* 2015). American pharmaceutical companies consider New Zealand to be hostile ground and one of the most restrictive markets in the world. Unable to meet their sales and profit targets, they argue it was becoming increasingly difficult to keep investments or even a presence in New Zealand. Given that New Zealand does not have a research-based pharmaceutical industry (Neuwelt *et al.* 2015) such threats are likely to have a minimal impact.

To summarise here, pharmaceutical companies have been able to exert influence over UK drug regulation through threats to the UK economy by withdrawing drug research, development and manufacturing facilities. Corporate bias is an ongoing issue in decision-making, compromising the ability of UK drug regulation agencies to exercise resistance against pharmaceutical companies. In New Zealand, the state drug buying agency is at an arms-length from the state, as governments cannot interfere with its decision-making processes. In addition, drug companies have limited leverage as they do not have a research base in New Zealand (Neuwelt *et al.* 2015). New Zealand then, has a greater possibility of resisting the expansion of pharmaceutical markets.

## Ideological resistance and alternative therapies

Resistance to pharmaceuticals takes place at a level of understanding about the causes of disease, the identification of those causes and their treatments. These are differences in terms of ontology, or what we think the world is made up of, and epistemology or how we think we can know about the world. As a shorthand I will refer simply to ideological differences, using ideology in the sense of a system of ideas. In this section, I will discuss the case of homeopathy to indicate the basis on which alternative medicines may act as a means of resistance to pharmaceuticalised governance.

Most people take alternative treatment, or attend an alternative therapist, for chronic conditions that are not life-threatening. Alternative therapeutic approaches often eschew pharmaceuticals, instead offering treatments that are not based on synthesised chemicals. The rise in the popularity of alternative health has variously been seen as a challenge to the dominance of the medical profession, an example of the post-modern condition and a sign of a fascination with New Age mythologies. As I noted in Chapter 1, I trained in an alternative therapeutic approach, osteopathy, in the UK. As such, I have a particular view on the place of alternative therapies in society, which is shaped by my experience training and practising as an osteopath. In terms of the patients I saw, I perceived most of them as trying out osteopathy because they had some problem (usually musculoskeletal, such as back pain) that was not going away and for which they had yet to find much help.

A problem in defining what alternative medicine means is that what is perceived to be alternative at one time may not be perceived as alternative at another, and even at the same time people differ in their views about what is alternative and what is orthodox. One useful definition states that 'the distinguishing feature of alternative therapies is their marginal standing in relation to the medical establishment and the health care system rather than any common content' (Baggott 1994: 33). This marginal standing is seen in their lack of access to state benefits, both in state subsidies of treatment costs and in the education of practitioners; their lack of access to hospitals; and the absence, or near absence, of legislation that allows those who practise the therapy to regulate its use. Clashes between orthodox and alternative medicine are likely to be over who has access to state funds, who has the right to control particular therapeutic techniques, and what standard should be used to provide credibility or legitimacy to a particular therapeutic approach (Dew 2000).

In the nineteenth century, homeopathy in particular posed a threat to the orthodox medicine of the time, gaining fashionable status and community support in Britain (Nicholls 1988), Australia (Willis 1983) and the US (Kaufman 1971). Many highly educated and orthodox practitioners abandoned regular medicine to take up homeopathy. In the US, homeopaths were generally receiving higher fees for their services, and had more successful practices than their orthodox colleagues. It is estimated that 10 per cent of medical practitioners in the US practised homeopathy at the start of the twentieth century (Berliner 1984). Homeopaths established the first national medical organisation in the US, the American Institute of Homeopathy, to regulate its members and ensure standards of education.

Homeopathy did not just provide a challenge to orthodox practitioners over custom, but more profoundly provided an ideological challenge. The principles of homeopathic practice and its understandings of disease and treatment were, and still are, completely at odds with conventional medical practice. Samuel Hahnemann, who developed the therapeutic approach of homeopathy, based treatment on three principles. The first is that the selection of the remedy for a patient is in accordance with the law of similars. The law of similars basically means that the remedy selected would reproduce the symptoms that the patient has in a healthy person. The second is the use of a minimum dose. Remedies are made up through a process of succussion and titration. Succussion is where the preparation is vigorously shaken in order to achieve an increase in the potency of the preparation. Titration is a process of serially diluting the preparation. What seems to be a paradox is that the more diluted the preparation, the more potent it is meant to be. With the process of dilution, many preparations would not have a single molecule of the substance in its final form. The third principle is that a single remedy should be used, not a combination. The goal of the prescriber is to match one particular remedy with the unique individual patient. Considering homeopathy from the perspective of conventional medicine one would assume that the preparations have no curative possibilities at all. How could they when they are so dilute? Many who practice homeopathy would suggest that the therapeutic process works at an energetic level, and not at a material level. Homeopathic understandings of the body, disease and therapeutics are at odds with orthodox approaches and challenge the focus on the use of toxic agents, like pharmaceuticals.

In nineteenth century America, there were 15,000 homeopathic practitioners, and homeopaths had the same legal status as regular medical practitioners (Coulter 1984). But in the early twentieth century homeopathy went into decline. In 1900, there were 22 homeopathic medical schools, but by 1923 there were only two. By the late 1950s, there were only 100 homeopathic physicians left in the US.

At times it is claimed that the decline of homeopathy was due to the triumph of scientific medicine, but it was rather the result of more complex cultural and social processes. For example, medical profession apologists have argued that the discovery of sulphonamides in 1935 foreshadowed the demise of homeopathy (Beaven 1989). Sulphonamides, in this argument, are considered to be the first recognised pharmaceutical treatment of the modern pharmacopoeia. Accounts along these lines fail to recognise that the decline of homeopathy occurred before medicine had any therapeutic capacity that would be regarded by contemporary standards as effective. Homeopathy was well in decline before the discovery of sulphonamides. The demise occurred when orthodox medicine was far from scientific, and was anything but therapeutic. Cultural changes in the perception of science and technology, changes in the therapeutic relationship with moves to hospital-based medicine, and the weakening of homeopathy due to internal struggles, all played a part in the decline of homeopathy (see Kaufman 1971, for an in-depth analysis of these processes). Phillip Nicholls notes that the stress on the unique features of each patient to find the specific remedy for that patient went against the need for high patient turnover, as the process of identifying that remedy could require a lengthy consultation (Nicholls 1988).

Since the 1950s, there has been a limited revival in interest in homeopathy in the US. In 1980, Arizona passed a homeopathic licensing law, followed in 1983 by Nevada (Coulter 1984). The revival has also been a commercial one, with homeopathic remedies widely available for sale in pharmacists and chemists.

Homeopathy is only one example of a therapeutic approach that challenges pharmaceutical-based therapies. Other therapies may use heterodox approaches that are not easily aligned with orthodox science. Some musculoskeletal approaches, such as some forms of osteopathy, may have vitalist principles, basing treatment on the existence of an invisible, vital element in the body, an energy, which the treatment attempts to appeal to. Some therapies may draw on different epistemologies and ontologies related to particular cultures, such as Ayurvedic medicine and traditional Chinese medicine and so on. As we saw in Chapter 5, householders are quite happy to mix up these different therapeutic approaches, and use therapies in novel ways that may combine pharmaceuticals with acupuncture, herbal remedies, body therapies and so on. Therefore, alternative approaches may be additional approaches, or pharmaceutical-based approaches may be additional to alternative and folk remedy approaches. Householders are less troubled by the political status of approaches as orthodox or unorthodox. Alternative approaches may, in addition, be conceptualised in ways that go beyond physiological responses, as people may gain a sense of well-being from using alternative approaches that link to their sense of identity (Sointu 2006).

Adherents of alternative therapeutic practices resist pharmaceuticalised governance as they make little use of pharmaceuticals as a therapeutic solution. Further, the principles that alternative therapies are grounded in may challenge the very basis for pharmaceutical solutions. Their success in the market place may even draw resources away from pharmaceuticals.

## Concluding comments

In this chapter, I have explored some avenues of resistance to pharmaceuticalisation and pharmaceuticalised governance, noting that it can occur at an individual, institutional and ideological level. Foucault argues that wherever there is power, there is resistance (Foucault 1978). There are other forms and means of resistance that I have not discussed in this chapter, such as resistance from health practitioners themselves who are concerned about the problem of medicalising what are in fact social problems in their patients (Dew *et al.* 2005), and insurance companies and hospital managers who want to reduce the costs of drugs to increase their profits or limit their expenses. Identifying forms of resistance to pharmaceuticalised governance provides a more nuanced picture of the role of pharmaceuticals in contemporary society, but resistance is of quite a limited nature.

Individuals resist pharmaceuticals, but I would suggest only around the margins. Resistance tends to be limited to modifying particular regimes, or trying to stay away from pharmaceuticals as much as possible. But the forces of pharmaceuticalisation noted in Chapter 3 mean more people going on medications to treat chronic conditions or to try to avoid future disease. In acute situations, pharmaceuticals will often be turned to as a solution. There are undoubtedly exceptions, such as people who refuse medications altogether, but these, I would suggest, are rare. It is not that pharmaceuticals dominate all aspects of our lives, but pharmaceuticals do remain a dominant form of therapeutic intervention.

Institutional or state resistance to pharmaceuticals is also muted. Even in the case of New Zealand, where the state drug buying agency can take an adversarial stance, state expenditure on pharmaceuticals continues to increase. State resistance is more around best value for money rather than any challenge to pharmaceuticalised governance.

At an ideological level, alternative therapeutic approaches can be in strong opposition to pharmaceuticals as a therapeutic approach. However, although individual alternative health practitioners may take an oppositional stance, and some of their patients may align with this, I would suggest that most patients take a pragmatic approach, and continue to rely on or use pharmaceuticals when they see fit. In addition to that, by definition, alternative therapies are marginalised in the health care system. The resistance to pharmaceuticalised governance is, in many ways, a sign of its strength.

## References

Abraham, J. (2009). Partial progress: Governing the pharmaceutical industry and the NHS, 1948–2008. *Journal of Health Politics Policy and Law* 34: 931–977.

American Psychiatric Association. (1968). *Diagnostic and Statistical Manual of Mental Disorders, Second Edition: DSM-II.* Washington, DC: American Psychiatric Association.

Baggott, R. (1994). *Health and Health Care in Britain.* Basingstoke: Macmillan.

Beaven, D. (1989). Alternative medicine a cruel hox – your money and your life? *New Zealand Medical Journal* 102: 416–417.

Begg, E., Sidwell, A., Gardiner, S. and Scott, R. (2003). The sorry saga of the statins in New Zealand – pharmacopolitics versus patient care. *New Zealand Medical Journal* 116 (1170): U360.

Bell, K. (2010). Cancer survivorship, mor(t)ality and lifestyle discourses on cancer prevention. *Sociology of Health and Illness* 32 (3): 349–364.

Berliner, H. (1984). Scientific medicine since Flexner. In: *Alternative Medicines: Popular and Policy Perspectives* (ed. J.W. Salmon), 30–56. New York: Tavistock Press.

Blackman, L. (2012). *Immaterial Bodies: Affect, Embodiment, Mediation.* London: Sage.

Britten, N., Riley, R. and Morgan, M. (2010). Resisting psychotropic medicines: A synthesis of qualitative studies of medicine-taking. *Advances in Psychiatric Treatment* 16: 207–218.

Broom, A. (2000). Boundary work: The construction of boundaries between 'alternative' and 'conventional' cancer treatments in New Zealand. Master thesis. University of Canterbury, Christchurch.

Broom, A. and Tovey, P. (2008). Exploring the temporal dimension in cancer patients' experiences of nonbiomedical therapeutics. *Qualitative Health Research* 18: 1650–1661.

Brown, K. (2017). Medical trial reveals Herceptin survival rate. *Radio New Zealand* www.radionz.co.nz/news/national/345704/medical-trial-reveals-herceptin-survival-rate (accessed 14 December 2017).

Brown, P. and Calnan, M. (2010). Braving a faceless new world? Conceptualizing trust in the pharmaceutical industry and its products. *Health* 16: 57–75.

Calnan, M., Hashem, F. and Brown, P. (2017). Still elegantly muddling through? NICE and uncertainty in decision making about the rationing of expensive medicines in England. *International Journal of Health Services* 47: 571–594.

Chamberlain, K., Madden, H., Gabe, J., Dew, K. and Norris, P. (2011). Forms of resistance to medication within New Zealand households. *Medische Anthroplogie* 23 (2): 299–308.

Collin, J. (2016). On social plasticity: The transformative power of pharmaceuticals on health, nature and identity. *Sociology of Health and Illness* 38: 73–89.

Coulter, H. (1984). Homeopathy. In: *Alternative Medicines: Popular and Policy Perspectives* (ed. J.W. Salmon), 57–79. New York: Tavistock Press.

Cunningham, A.J., Phillips, C., Lockwood, G.A., Hedley, D.W. and Edmonds, C.V. (2000). Association of involvement in psychological self-regulation with longer survival in patients with metastatic cancer: An exploratory study. *Advances in Mind-Body Medicine* 16 (4): 276–286.

Dew, K. (2000). Apostasy to orthodoxy: Debates before a Commission of Inquiry into chiropractic. *Sociology of Health and Illness* 22: 1310–1330.

Dew, K. and Davis, A. (2014). Limits to neo-liberal reforms in the health sector: The case of pharmaceutical management in New Zealand. *International Journal of Health Services Volume* 44: 137–153.

Dew, K., Dowell, A., McLeod, D., Collings, S. and Bushnell, J. (2005). 'This glorious twilight zone of uncertainty': Mental health consultations in general practice in New Zealand. *Social Science and Medicine* 61 (6): 1189–1200.

Dew, K., Signal, L., Stairmand, J., Simpson, A. and Sarfati, D. (Forthcoming). Cancer care decision-making and treatment consent: An observational study of patients' and clinicians' rights. *Journal of Sociology*.

Dowell, J. and Hudson, H. (1997). A qualitative study of medication-taking behaviour in primary care. *Family Practice* 14: 369–375.

Fainzang, S. (2017). *Self-Medication and Society: Mirages of Autonomy*. Abingdon: Routledge.

Foucault, M. (1978). *The History of Sexuality: An Introduction*. Allen Lane: London.

Gabe, J., Chamberlain, K., Norris, P., Dew, K., Madden, H. and Hodgetts, D. (2012). The debate about the funding of Herceptin: A case study of 'countervailing powers'. *Social Science and Medicine* 75 (12): 2353–2361.

Hare, E. (1962). Masturbatory insanity: The history of an idea. *Journal of Mental Science* 108: 2–25.

Healy, D. (2006). Manufacturing consensus. *Culture, Medicine and Psychiatry* 30: 135–156.

Hodgetts, D., Young-Hauser, A., Chamberlain, K., Gabe, J., Dew, K. and Norris, P. (2017). Pharmaceuticalisation in the city. *Urban Studies* 54 (15): 3542–3559.

Hök, J., Forss, A., Falkenberg, T. and Tishelman, C. (2009). What is an exceptional cancer trajectory?: Multiple stakeholder perspectives on cancer trajectories in relation to complementary and alternative medicine use. *Integrative Cancer Therapies* 8 (2): 153–163.

Kaufman, M. (1971). *Homeopathy in America: The Rise and Fall of a Medical Heresy*. Baltimore: Johns Hopkins University Press.

Martin, E. (2006). The pharmaceutical person. *BioSocieties* 1: 273–287.

Moore, D., Scott, A. and Walker, M. (1996). The great debate about reference pricing of pharmaceuticals. In: *Healthy Incentives: Canadian Health Reform in an International Context* (eds W. McArthur, C. Ramsay and M. Walker), 101–108. Vancouver: The Fraser Institute.

Neuwelt, P., Gleeson, D. and Mannering, B. (2015). Patently obvious: A public health analysis of pharmaceutical industry statements on the Trans-Pacific-Partnership international trade agreement. *Critical Public Health* 26: 159–172.

Nicholls, P. (1988). *Homoeopathy and the Medical Profession*. London: Croom Helm.

Pound, P., Britten, N., Morgan, M., Yardley, L., Pope, C., Daker-White, G. and Campbell, R. (2005). Resisting medicines: A synthesis of qualitative studies of medicine taking. *Social Science and Medicine* 61 (1): 133–155.

Sointu, E. (2006). The search for wellbeing in alternative and complementary health practices. *Sociology of Health and Illness* 28: 330–349.

The New Zealand Herald. (2010). WikiLeaks cable: No quick fix for pharmaceutical market. *The New Zealand Herald* (19 December).

Willis, E. (1983). *Medical Dominance: The Division of Labour in Australian Healthcare*. Sydney: George Allen and Unwin.

Woodfield, A. (2001). Augmenting reference pricing of pharmaceuticals with strategic cross-product agreements. *Pharmacoeconomics* 19: 365–377.

Zhong, L. (2003). Negotiating the price and subsidy for prescription drugs: The case of lipitor in New Zealand. Palmerson North: Management Research, Massey University.

# 13 Drug entanglements and governance

The astonishing economic and popular success of pharmaceuticals as a therapeutic intervention places pharmaceuticals in a unique space in contemporary society. A consequence of pharmaceutical success is that many aspects of our lives are governed through pharmaceuticals. How are we to understand the extraordinary presence of pharmaceuticals in our lives and their impact on so many institutions?

I suggest that a starting place is the connection between pharmaceuticals and economic organisation. In terms of a therapeutic approach, pharmaceuticals appear to be just about the ideal one to align with capitalism. I suggest that there is a powerful elective affinity between them. Max Weber introduced the concept of elective affinity to sociology and used it most famously in his book *The Protestant Ethic and the Spirit of Capitalism* (Weber 1976). Weber claimed an elective affinity between certain forms of Protestantism and capitalism. It was not that one caused the other, but that they influenced one another in a reciprocal relationship, and this in turn had consequences for the historical development of both capitalism and Protestantism (Howe 1978). The mass production of pharmaceuticals occurs as the technological capacities and distribution capabilities of capitalism develop. A therapeutic approach that requires standardised diagnoses and treatment aligns with the mass marketing of pharmaceuticals and with the demands of capitalism. The entanglement of the medical profession in these developments connects with a therapeutic regime that requires the control of the therapeutic agent because of its toxicity. The use of pharmaceuticals additionally aligns with the ideals of a more efficient health care delivery system. With standardised diagnoses and treatments, and shorter consultation times, health care can be delivered more efficiently.

The expansion of a drug industry aligning with capitalist goals of expanding markets and higher rates of consumption comes up against state concerns for safety and ensuring benefit for the population. As the drug industry cannot be trusted to determine safety, seen in such drug disasters as Thalidomide and Vioxx, then the drug industry needs to be regulated. A technology of regulation is readily at hand in the form of the randomised controlled trial (RCT). Although there is some resistance to the imposition of expensive regulatory mechanisms on the drug industry, the use of RCTs has a number of outcomes that further strengthen the industry as a whole.

One outcome is that RCTs subsequently became the centrepiece of the Evidence-Based Medicine (EBM) movement. A form of assessment that is designed to test the safety and efficacy of drugs now becomes the form of assessment that every therapeutic regime must pass through if it is to gain legitimacy. But entire therapeutic approaches are not based on the assumptions of the RCT. The example of homeopathy illustrates that. In its classical form its diagnoses and treatments are not standardised. It can never be double-blinded as an expert has to decide upon a specific remedy for the particular patient, so it can never gain credibility.

Not only do pharmaceuticals provide the medical profession with its most potent therapeutic products, but they shape the way in which medical professionals are assessed and overseen. This results from the interlinking of tests for efficacy and safety with EBM and with the requirements of medical practitioners to conform to evidence-based guidelines. To fail to conform to recommendations based on EBM, which are in turn based on the RCT, which in turn strongly favours pharmaceuticals, is to be identified as potentially deviant. Medical practitioners are now firmly governed through pharmaceuticals. It is not the case that the medical professionals simply opt to use pharmaceuticals. Pharmaceuticalised governance limits and constrains the options that are available to them.

What started as a means of testing toxic substances that are used for therapeutic effect that is, the use of clinical trials, has now provided an incontestable legitimation to the use of drugs as the major therapeutic approach. As the medical profession embeds its therapeutic approach firmly in pharmaceuticals and the trial of the RCT, it can facilitate its dominance over other therapeutic modalities. The drug industry is not threatened at all by challenges from alternative therapeutic approaches as it is so firmly linked to the medical profession and to the RCT. Once the RCT comes to dominate it changes what we see. We no longer believe what we see before our eyes, such as the impact of a sacroiliac adjustment I noted in Chapter 1; we can only trust what has been validated by the RCT. The 'we' used here might not apply to you personally, but it applies to a system of legitimation that affects us all.

There is then a powerful affinity between the goal of delivering an efficient health care system, professionalising tactics of the medical profession, the capitalist orientation of pharmaceutical companies, and the form of therapeutic legitimation that has developed.

The drug industry and pharmaceuticals have shaped capitalism. Developments in intellectual property to protect the profits of drug companies enter into trade agreements across the world. The desire of drug companies to have unregulated access to markets drives endeavours to limit the sovereignty of nation-states. The powerful imagery of granting people access to needed medications has the potential to act as a lever against state sovereignty like no other product. The drug industry has other tactics, such as threats to developed nations that they will withdraw their manufacturing base from those nations.

The drug industry can have a strong impact on the life chances of millions of people in the Global South by neglecting to undertake research on tropical

diseases. Challenges posed to the reputation of the drug industry by the existence of drug-treatable disease in the Global South have led to changes in the
development and distribution of pharmaceuticals. Philanthro-capitalism is an
important form in the development and distribution of drugs, circumventing
international charities and governments in the delivery of programmes. The
focus of philanthro-capitalism on single-disease projects draws attention away
from the social organisation of poverty and misery, and social and political
solutions to that poverty. Interventions in the Global South that are focused on
access to pharmaceuticals may act to obscure other social problems from the
view of philanthropists and policy makers, such as dangerous work practices
or malnutrition. Pharmaceuticals embedded within capitalist relations can play
a significant role in exacerbating health and social inequalities. On the one
hand this may lessen the chance of overmedication in the Global South, but on
the other it may expose users to more dangerous drug usage through unregulated markets or mean people miss out on life-saving or symptom relieving
drugs.

State interests can favour the promotion of pharmaceuticals. The state can
foster public health interventions aimed at the entire population, as with vaccines. The state can target particular population groups, as with the development
of guidelines and recommendations to promote cholesterol-lowering drugs. The
influence of population health perspectives focuses attention on how to prevent
future disease, so as to increase longevity, reduce morbidity and limit future
health care costs. An illustration of this is work to develop a polypill. This pill is
aimed at reducing cardiovascular disease. Trials have been undertaken on polypills that combine cholesterol-lowering drugs, blood pressure drugs and aspirin.
The concept is that everyone over a certain age, possibly 55, would take the pill
and that they would not need to see a doctor or have any monitoring in relation
to the pill (Viera 2017). This is a population health strategy. If it follows a
similar logic to the population health strategy of vaccinations everyone may be
compelled to take polypills to access state benefits. I would suggest that we are
likely to see further advances in drug-based population health approaches due to
powerful vested interests that would support such developments. It suits the
state, in that it can claim to be carrying out its pastoral care duties, taking care of
the population. Additionally, for the state, drug-based population health strategies may align with the goals of containing future health care costs, avoiding
hospitalisations from heart disease, and reducing productivity losses resulting
from worker illness. It suits medical professionals in that it provides powerful
legitimacy for its therapeutic approach. These strategies suit drug companies
who can reap the profits from such population health thinking.

Although a pharmaceutical approach to therapeutics has supported the dominance of the medical profession in the health care landscape, the medical profession loses some control as the drug industry expands its advertising and sales
activities into cyberspace. The new opportunities to market and sell directly to
consumers have the potential to fundamentally change the relationship between
patients, physicians and pharmaceuticals. Physicians may be taken out of the

loop, or patients may take information provided directly by drug companies into the health care consultation to influence the outcome. Cyberspace furthermore provides opportunities for a form of pharmacosociality, where people taking the same drugs can share their experiences. Drug users sharing experiences can alert people to a host of issues, such as off-label benefits or, alternatively, under-reported adverse drug reactions (ADRs).

The interweaving of cyberspace and pharmacosociality can produce new political subjects. Drug industry attempts to control the distribution of drugs and their prices in different nations promotes new political subjects. Buyers' clubs have formed to allow people from the Global North to avoid paying extortionate prices for drugs by allowing purchases of drugs at far lower cost in the Global South. Buyers' clubs therefore, act to undermine the profit gouging of drug companies under a banner of social justice (Quet 2018).

Commentators have raised many concerns about the way pharmaceuticals get on to the market and are used. Drugs play such a powerful role in society because they work. They save lives. This power enables manifold forms of pharmaceuticalised governance that is difficult to resist. All would be fine if we could trust those who manufacture drugs, but the science of pharmaceuticals can be a perversion of science (Merton 1973). In terms of drug development, concerns have been raised about the conduct of clinical trials. Only a very limited faith can be placed in clinical trials, despite the huge resources that go into them, and so the public is exposed to potential adverse reactions once drugs are on the market. Researchers have shown how drug companies highlight positive results about their product, conceal negative results, and lobby regulatory agencies and health professionals to expand the categories of disease for which drugs can be used and the population of potential drug users.

The dominating role of pharmaceuticals in society along with concerns about their expense and toxicity has led to the development of various agencies to oversee, regulate and shape pharmaceutical consumption. Not only do pharmaceuticals provide people with opportunities to find relief from symptoms and disease, they create disease and cause death. Pharmacovigilance agencies, noting the failure to report most adverse reactions once drugs are on the market, explore new ways of identifying problem drugs, such as checking patient websites to identify from patient stories indications of adverse reactions to drugs (Medawar *et al.* 2002). Drug regulatory agencies, which developed and transformed over many decades, can at various times or in different places align with and facilitate drug company access to markets, or attempt to temper and limit that access. Efforts to respond to the danger and potential of drugs have generated new institutions. Advocacy organisations, such as Health Action International, have formed to expose unethical practices of pharmaceutical companies, and patient activist groups have been mobilised to support the biomedical research for medicines that pharmaceutical companies profit from (O'Donovan 2007). Drug regulatory agencies, drug buying agencies, research companies, pharmacovigilance agencies, philanthropic agencies, lobbying groups and drug consumer support groups have all been spawned.

At the level of everyday experience we are exposed to a barrage of drug advertising through all media, and through our everyday activities. Pharmaceuticals permeate our everyday lives. We are confronted with images related to drugs on television and computers, on the streets with billboard advertising and the stocks of drugs in pharmacies and supermarkets. Pharmaceutical concerns enter into our conversations with family, friends and colleagues. Households, however, are uncontrolled spaces of pharmaceuticalised governance. The inexorable processes of pharmaceuticalisation occurring at a societal level are transformed in the everyday practices of people in their households. Societal efforts are made to standardise medication, who prescribes them, what they are prescribed for, at what dose and for how long. But in everyday life these standardised practices can be undermined. Therapeutic actions are not subject in any simplistic way to a dominant mode of understanding. Drugs are spread throughout these spaces. They may be resisted at times, and advice may be modified. They may be combined with other therapeutic approaches. But drugs dominate in this space too, and the moral compulsion to consume is strongly felt, even if the drugs are seen as a necessary evil and not embraced.

The routines of pharmaceutical consumption change relationships between people and places. Family members oversee each other's consumption of drugs. Household spaces are used as reminders of a required routine. Householders take on responsibilities for others to ensure they conform and act in morally appropriate ways as good pharmaceuticalised citizens. Pharmaceuticals bring about changes in relationships, some obvious, some subtle. Drug formulations can enhance stigma, as with people who have to take drugs in front of peers, or reduce stigma, as with antiretroviral therapy destigmatising intimate relations between serodiscordant people. In the process of engaging with drugs, people's identities are transformed and with psychotropic drugs their sense of self can change. The kinds of beings we see ourselves as can change, from thinking agents with free will to a body of chemical reactions that can be influenced by pharmaceuticals.

Pharmaceuticals can act, in tandem with new diagnostic categories, to fundamentally change the meaning and sense of taken-for-granted concepts. Pharmaceuticals alter understandings of normality. Proto-diseases mean we are never in a non-diseased state. New identities are created around diseases of risk as drug-based preventive measures are promoted, which identify one's physiology as a liability for life. Pharmaceuticals to enhance our capacities, to make us better than normal, challenge or change what is conceived of as normal.

There is a tension in pharmaceuticalised governance between the goals of standardising and normalising bodies and the goal of enhancing our biological capacities. Will we see a shift of resources to drugs that enhance our capabilities? Will we see cognitive enhancing drugs and stimulants subsidised by the state for workers who need to work long hours in challenging environments? Will we see state subsidisation of menstrual suppression drugs to make it easier for women in the military to go into battle? Students may feel compelled to take cognitive enhancing drugs to improve their academic performance. Those who resist such measures or cannot afford to access the drugs may have more limited opportunities in life.

Pharmaceuticalised governance refers to the ways pharmaceuticals shape our conduct and ways of being. It is not just the profit motive that ultimately shapes forms of pharmaceuticalised governance. Capitalist motives are crucial for creating the particular form of the drug market and how it operates, but interactional forces, the forces of everyday life, are entangled in ways that shape our conduct and drug taking behaviours. How drugs are prescribed by health professionals and responded to by patients is shaped by powerful interactional forces leading, for example, to the underreporting of ADRs. We are subjected by other organisations, professionals and social demands to consume pharmaceuticals. Pharmaceuticals shape us as subjects and shape broader social arrangements. The influences shaping particular forms of pharmaceuticalised governance are myriad. I suggest that we are in the midst of an accumulating process entangling many social practices with pharmaceuticals.

Pharmaceuticalised governance can be understood as operating through interacting domains. In the home, standardising procedures are broken down as householders adapt, combine or reject protocols, guidelines and recommendations, providing a space of resistance to governance. Relations of care may dominate over concerns for profit. But pharmaceuticals are ever present and close to hand. They are readily consumed. Relations of care can invoke different forms of governance, with close monitoring of others, badgering and organising the house around routines of pharmaceutical consumption.

In the space of the clinic of the orthodox medical practitioner, pharmaceuticals are the dominant therapeutic modality. Doctors readily prescribe. Patients may resist, but resistance is constrained by the powerful structural forces that make pharmaceuticals the focus of therapeutics and shape the actions of medical professionals to conform to the requirements of EBM and its RCT hierarchy. In the clinic these powerful forces are entangled with interactional forces that work to dampen conflict as practitioners and patients work to protect each other's face.

For the state, expenditure on pharmaceuticals and the promotion of their use can be seen as an outcome of pastoral concerns to protect the population but also attempts to control the population and to prevent further expense from future disease. These forces of pharmaceutical promotion are in tension with concerns about the expense of drugs, especially new ones, and their safety.

At an international level, pharmaceuticals hold the promise of providing relief from deadly or debilitating diseases, promoting efforts from states, non-governmental organisations and philanthro-capitalists to advance their use. Such a focus can draw attention away from the social determinants of disease, such as poverty, malnutrition and poor working conditions.

The influences on increasing levels of pharmaceutical consumption are socially, culturally and politically complex. There are shifts in people's expectations about illness and how it should be responded to, there are technological developments that open up new possibilities for treatment, there are changes to the regulatory oversight of pharmaceuticals, and states develop new polices on the availability and subsidisation of pharmaceuticals. Debates and practices around pharmaceuticals are permeated with dilemmas. We might desire an increase in access to drugs though this can expose us to the dangers of their toxicity. We might desire drug companies to be profitable to support the labour market though this may incite a focus on drugs being developed for the wealthy Global North and so exacerbate health inequalities. We may desire innovative practices though this may conflict with regulatory regimes.

Noting the variability in pharmaceuticalised governance across nation-states and amongst social groups it is worth exploring these issues in more depth, to consider ways in which pharmaceuticals shape identity, exacerbate or mitigate social inequalities and act as mediators of broader shifts in social policy and economic organisation.

How we act in relation to pharmaceuticals, whether we choose to seek out drug-based therapies to deal with health problems, whether we support regulation to control the activities of drug companies, whether we give to charities that look to pharmaceuticals to respond to social troubles, depends on what we find convincing, at this particular time in this particular set of circumstances. Is the extensive hold of pharmaceuticalised governance inevitable? It appears to be. It is possible to envisage other forms of therapeutic governance, based on non-pharmaceutical approaches or where pharmaceuticals are used to supplement some other dominant form of therapy. Perhaps it is relatively easy for me to consider such possibilities, given my training in an alternative approach and because of my own experiences. However, I am not aware of any developments that would make me think that a challenge to pharmaceuticalised governance is likely.

Pharmaceuticalised governance takes different shapes, but within a global context of increasing pharmaceuticalisation. Pharmaceutical solutions are inextricably entangled in our everyday lives.

## References

Howe, R.H. (1978). Max Weber's elective affinities: Sociology within the bounds of pure reason. *American Journal of Sociology* 84 (2): 366–385.

Medawar, C., Herxheimer, A., Bell, A. and Jofre, S. (2002). Paroxetine, panorama and user reporting of ADRs: Consumer intelligence matters in clinical practice and post-marketing drug surveillance. *International Journal of Risk and Safety in Medicine* 15: 161–169.

Merton, R.K. (1973). *The Sociology of Science: Theoretical and Empirical Investigations.* Chicago and London: The University of Chicago Press.

O'Donovan, O. (2007). Corporate colonization of health activism? Irish health advocacy organization's modes of engagement with pharmaceutical corporations. *International Journal of Health Services* 37 (4): 711–733.

Quet, M. (2018). Pharmaceutical capitalism and its logistics: access to hepatitis C treatment. *Theory, Culture and Society* 35 (2): 67–89.

Viera, A. (2017). Whatever happened to the polypill. *British Medical Journal* 356: j1474.

Weber, M. (1976). *The Protestant Ethic and the Spirit of Capitalism*: George Allen and Unwin.

# Index

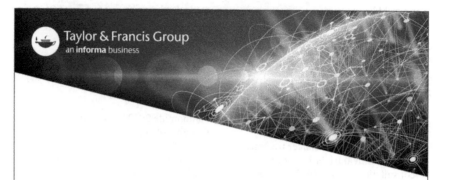

# Taylor & Francis eBooks

www.taylorfrancis.com

A single destination for eBooks from Taylor & Francis
with increased functionality and an improved user
experience to meet the needs of our customers.

90,000+ eBooks of award-winning academic content in
Humanities, Social Science, Science, Technology, Engineering,
and Medical written by a global network of editors and authors.

## TAYLOR & FRANCIS EBOOKS OFFERS:

A streamlined
experience for
our library
customers

A single point
of discovery
for all of our
eBook content

Improved
search and
discovery of
content at both
book and
chapter level

## REQUEST A FREE TRIAL
support@taylorfrancis.com

Milton Keynes UK
Ingram Content Group UK Ltd.
UKHW040056071024
449327UK00019B/591